Advances in Glaucoma Treatment

Advances in Glaucoma Treatment

Editor

Georgios Labiris

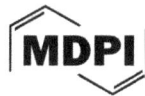

Basel • Beijing • Wuhan • Barcelona • Belgrade • Novi Sad • Cluj • Manchester

Editor
Georgios Labiris
University Hospital of Alexandroupolis
Alexandroupolis
Greece

Editorial Office
MDPI
St. Alban-Anlage 66
4052 Basel, Switzerland

This is a reprint of articles from the Special Issue published online in the open access journal *Journal of Clinical Medicine* (ISSN 2077-0383) (available at: https://www.mdpi.com/journal/jcm/special_issues/Advances_Glaucoma_Treatment).

For citation purposes, cite each article independently as indicated on the article page online and as indicated below:

Lastname, A.A.; Lastname, B.B. Article Title. *Journal Name* **Year**, *Volume Number*, Page Range.

ISBN 978-3-7258-0199-2 (Hbk)
ISBN 978-3-7258-0200-5 (PDF)
doi.org/10.3390/books978-3-7258-0200-5

© 2024 by the authors. Articles in this book are Open Access and distributed under the Creative Commons Attribution (CC BY) license. The book as a whole is distributed by MDPI under the terms and conditions of the Creative Commons Attribution-NonCommercial-NoDerivs (CC BY-NC-ND) license.

Contents

Yusaku Miura and Ken Fukuda
Comparison of Different Procedures in a Combination of Ab Interno Microhook Trabeculotomy
and Cataract Surgery
Reprinted from: *J. Clin. Med.* **2022**, *11*, 738, doi:10.3390/jcm11030738 1

Luigi Fontana and Alberto Neri
Microcatheter–Assisted Circumferential Trabeculotomy in Primary Congenital Glaucoma:
Long-Term Clinical Outcomes
Reprinted from: *J. Clin. Med.* **2022**, *11*, 414, doi:10.3390/jcm11020414 8

**Felix Mathias Wagner, Alexander Karl-Georg Schuster, Franz Grehn, Lukas Urbarek,
Norbert Pfeiffer, Julia Verena Stingl and Esther Maria Hoffmann**
Twenty-Years of Experience in Childhood Glaucoma Surgery
Reprinted from: *J. Clin. Med.* **2021**, *10*, 5720, doi:10.3390/jcm10245720 18

**Hiromitsu Onoe, Kazuyuki Hirooka, Mikio Nagayama, Atsushi Hirota, Hideki Mochizuki,
Takeshi Sagara, et al.**
The Efficacy, Safety and Satisfaction Associated with Switching from Brinzolamide 1% and
Brimonidine 0.1% to a Fixed Combination of Brinzolamide 1% and Brimonidine 0.1% in
Glaucoma Patients
Reprinted from: *J. Clin. Med.* **2021**, *10*, 5228, doi:10.3390/jcm10225228 29

Pei-Yao Chang, Jiun-Yi Wang, Jia-Kang Wang, Tzu-Lun Huang and Yung-Ray Hsu
Comparison of Treatment Outcomes of Selective Laser Trabeculoplasty for Primary Open-Angle
Glaucoma and Pseudophakic Primary Angle-Closure Glaucoma Receiving Maximal Medical
Therapy
Reprinted from: *J. Clin. Med.* **2021**, *10*, 2853, doi:10.3390/jcm10132853 35

**Antonio Maria Fea, Martina Menchini, Alessandro Rossi, Chiara Posarelli,
Lorenza Malinverni and Michele Figus**
Early Experience with the New XEN63 Implant in Primary Open-Angle Glaucoma Patients:
Clinical Outcomes
Reprinted from: *J. Clin. Med.* **2021**, *10*, 1628, doi:10.3390/jcm10081628 46

**Kee Sup Park, Kyoung Nam Kim, Jaeyoung Kim, Yeon Hee Lee, Sung Bok Lee
and Chang-sik Kim**
Effects of Miosis on Anterior Chamber Structure in Glaucoma Implant Surgery
Reprinted from: *J. Clin. Med.* **2021**, *10*, 1017, doi:10.3390/jcm10051017 57

Ke-Hao Huang, Ching-Long Chen, Da-Wen Lu, Jiann-Torng Chen and Yi-Hao Chen
Outcomes of Small Size Ahmed Glaucoma Valve Implantation in Asian Chronic Angle-Closure
Glaucoma
Reprinted from: *J. Clin. Med.* **2021**, *10*, 813, doi:10.3390/jcm10040813 67

**Aristeidis Konstantinidis, Eirini-Kanella Panagiotopoulou, Georgios D. Panos,
Haris Sideroudi, Aysel Mehmet and Georgios Labiris**
The Effect of Antiglaucoma Procedures (Trabeculectomy vs. Ex-PRESS Glaucoma Drainage
Implant) on the Corneal Biomechanical Properties
Reprinted from: *J. Clin. Med.* **2021**, *10*, 802, doi:10.3390/jcm10040802 80

Joanna Konopińska, Anna Byszewska, Emil Saeed, Zofia Mariak and Marek Rękas
Phacotrabeculectomy versus Phaco with Implantation of the Ex-PRESS Device: Surgical and
Refractive Outcomes—A Randomized Controlled Trial
Reprinted from: *J. Clin. Med.* **2021**, *10*, 424, doi:10.3390/jcm10030424 89

Katarzyna Konieczka and Josef Flammer
Treatment of Glaucoma Patients with Flammer Syndrome
Reprinted from: *J. Clin. Med.* **2021**, *10*, 4227, doi:10.3390/jcm10184227 . . . . **101**

Article

Comparison of Different Procedures in a Combination of Ab Interno Microhook Trabeculotomy and Cataract Surgery

Yusaku Miura and Ken Fukuda *

Department of Ophthalmology and Visual Science, Kochi Medical School, Kochi University, Nankoku 783-8505, Japan; miurasaku@kochi-u.ac.jp
* Correspondence: k.fukuda@kochi-u.ac.jp; Tel.: +81-88880-2391

Abstract: The purpose of this study was to compare the clinical outcomes of ab interno microhook trabeculotomy (μLOT) before and after cataract surgery for the combination of μLOT and cataract surgery. This retrospective case series included 40 eyes that underwent μLOT combined with cataract surgery at Kochi University Hospital. Groups 1 (20 eyes) and 2 (20 eyes) included eyes that underwent μLOT before and after cataract surgery, respectively. The patient characteristics and clinical outcomes were also analyzed. The mean preoperative intraocular pressure (IOP) in Groups 1 and 2 (26.1 ± 12.2 mmHg and 20.6 ± 8.8 mmHg) was reduced significantly to 14.1 ± 3.3 mmHg and 12.9 ± 3.2 mmHg, respectively, at 5–7 months postoperatively. The median preoperative number of antiglaucoma medications in Groups 1 and 2 (4.0 and 3.5) also decreased significantly, to 2.5 and 1.0, respectively, at 5–7 months postoperatively. Postoperative hyphema with niveau formation in Groups 1 and 2 was observed in one eye (5.0%) and six eyes (30.0%), respectively. For the combination of μLOT and cataract surgery, performing μLOT before cataract surgery may be less likely to result in postoperative hyphema with niveau formation.

Keywords: minimally invasive glaucoma surgery (MIGS); microhook; hyphema; surgical efficacy; surgical complication

1. Introduction

Trabeculotomy (LOT) is performed in patients with mild to moderate glaucoma other than angle-closure glaucoma to reduce the intraocular pressure (IOP) by reducing the resistance to aqueous flow by incising the trabecular meshwork and the inner wall of the Schlemm canal [1–4]. Recently, minimally invasive glaucoma surgery (MIGS) has been reported as a safer and less traumatic ab interno surgical procedure [5–8]. Unlike conventional ab externo LOT using metal trabeculotomy, MIGS tends to involve minimal trauma with very little or no scleral dissection, minimal or no conjunctival manipulation, good safety, and rapid recovery [9]. Among MIGS, the microhook LOT (μLOT) reported by Tanito is especially easy and less time-consuming to perform because the tip of the hook is much smaller than that in the other gonio-surgery devices, and the intracameral manipulation of the hook is easier than in the other devices [10]. A recent study has revealed that μLOT is effective in reducing IOP especially in glaucoma patients with older age, steroid-induced glaucoma, or developmental glaucoma [11]. Another advantage of μLOT is that it does not require expensive devices [10]. However, a study of combined cataract surgery and μLOT reported postoperative hyphema with niveau formation in 41% of cases [12], while another study of combined cataract surgery and Kahook dual blade categorized as MIGS reported no postoperative hyphema with niveau formation [13]. These studies utilized different surgical procedures and instruments. Hirabayashi et al. performed ab interno LOT using a Kahook dual blade before cataract surgery [13]. In contrast, Tanito et al. performed μLOT after cataract surgery; however, the reason for performing μLOT after and not before cataract surgery was not described [12]. Thus, it is not clear whether μLOT should be performed before or after cataract surgery. We hypothesized that the frequency of hyphema may vary depending on whether μLOT is performed before or after cataract surgery. Therefore, the present study compared μLOT before and after cataract surgery to determine if there were differences in clinical outcomes according to the timing of the cataract procedure.

2. Materials and Methods

2.1. Methods

Our study included patients with glaucoma who underwent μLOT before (Group 1) or after (Group 2) cataract surgery.

Most surgeries were performed by a single surgeon (Y.M.). Some surgeries were performed by four doctors supervised by Y.M. between April 2019 and June 2021 at Kochi University Hospital, Japan. We selected patients with early stage glaucoma who had not yet undergone surgery. All eyes included in this study had an open-angle and identifiable trabecular meshwork under gonioscopy. We excluded patients with angle-closure glaucoma, a postoperative follow-up of <5 months, or a history of glaucoma surgery. Data including age, sex, glaucoma type, IOP based on Goldmann applanation tonometry, number of antiglaucoma medications, best-corrected visual acuity (BCVA), surgical time, intraoperative and postoperative complications, and interventions for complications were collected from the medical charts.

2.2. Surgical Procedure

First, peribulbar anesthesia was performed in all eyes using a sub-Tenon injection of 2% lidocaine. In Group 1, μLOT was performed using the following procedure: viscoelastic material (1% sodium hyaluronate, Opegan Hi, Santen Pharmaceutical, Osaka, Japan) was injected into the anterior chamber (AC) through two corneal ports on the temporal side created using a 20-gauge microvitreoretinal (MVR) knife (Mani, Utsunomiya, Japan). Using a Hill surgical gonioprism (Ocular Instruments, Bellevue, WA, USA) to observe the angle opposite the corneal port, a microhook was inserted into the AC through the corneal port. The tip of the microhook was then inserted into the Schlemm's canal and moved circumferentially to incise the inner wall of the Schlemm's canal and trabecular meshwork over 2 clock hours (Figure 1). Using the same procedure, LOT was performed using a microhook inserted through another corneal port. That is, a trabecular meshwork totaling 120 degrees or more was incised. In Group 1, standard phacoemulsification with IOL implantation was performed through an additional temporal corneal 2.8 mm incision. In Group 2, μLOT was performed using the same procedure as described above after standard phacoemulsification with IOL implantation. After surgery, postoperative long-standing hyphema was treated with anterior chamber washout. Postoperative blood accumulation in the lens bag was treated using Nd:YAG laser capsulotomy to disperse the accumulated blood.

2.3. Outcome Measures

The primary outcome was the frequency of hyphema with niveau formation, which was defined as a hemorrhagic niveau of 0.5 mm or more at the inferior part of the anterior chamber. The secondary outcome was IOP measured 5–7 months after surgery. Surgical success was defined as: (1) $6 \leq IOP \leq 21$ and a reduction of more than 20% with or without antiglaucoma medications; (2) no loss of light perception; and (3) no additional glaucoma surgery. Transient IOP elevation within 1 month postoperatively was considered an IOP spike and was not classified as a surgical failure.

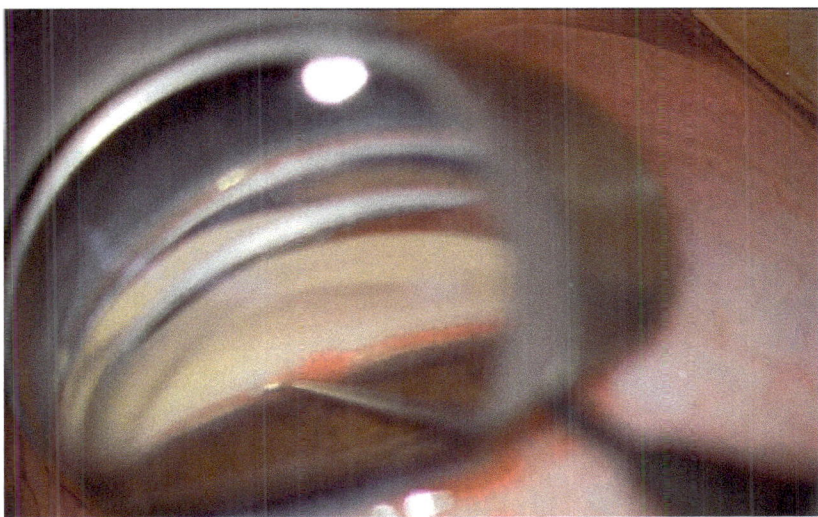

Figure 1. Intraoperative photograph of microhook ab interno trabeculotomy. Observation of the anterior-chamber angle using a Hill surgical gonioprism shows the trabecular meshwork and the process of cutting through the inner wall of Schlemm's canal circumferentially using the microhook inserted through a small corneal incision.

2.4. Statistical Analysis

BCVA was converted to the logarithm of the minimum angle of resolution (logMAR) for statistical analysis. Wilcoxon signed-rank tests were used to compare IOP, number of antiglaucoma medications, and BCVA values preoperatively and 5–7 months postoperatively. Wilcoxon rank-sum tests were used to evaluate the group differences between continuous variables. The incidence of complications was compared between the groups using Fisher exact tests. Statistical significance was set at $p < 0.05$. All data were entered into an Excel spreadsheet (Microsoft Corp., Redmond, WA, USA) and analyzed using Excel 2016 with the add-in software Statcel 4.

3. Results

This retrospective study included a total of 40 eyes from 31 patients who underwent surgery. Groups 1 and 2 comprised 20 eyes of 16 patients and 20 eyes of 15 patients, respectively. The patient characteristics are shown in Table 1. The two groups were well-matched for demographic characteristics.

The mean IOP in Group 1 decreased significantly, from 26.1 ± 12.2 mmHg at baseline to 14.1 ± 3.3 mmHg at 5–7 months postoperatively ($p = 0.000089$) (Table 2). Similarly, the mean IOP in Group 2 decreased significantly, from 20.6 ± 8.8 mmHg at baseline to 12.9 ± 3.2 mmHg at 5–7 months postoperatively ($p = 0.00014$). The mean (±SD) percentage of IOP reduction from baseline was 38.3% (±20.0) and 31.3% (±21.4) in Groups 1 and 2, respectively. The mean IOPs did not differ significantly between the two groups at baseline and 5–7 months postoperatively. The median number of antiglaucoma medications in Group 1 decreased significantly from 4.0 (3–5) at baseline to 2.5 (2–3) at 5–7 months postoperatively ($p = 0.0011$). Similarly, the median number of antiglaucoma medications in Group 2 also decreased significantly, from 3.5 (2–4.25) to 1.0 (0–3) ($p = 0.00048$). The median number of antiglaucoma medications did not differ significantly between the two groups at baseline and 5–7 months postoperatively. The mean best corrected visual acuity (BCVA) in Group 1 improved significantly from 0.27 ± 0.28 at baseline to −0.004 ± 0.18 at 5–7 months postoperatively ($p = 0.00032$). Similarly, the mean BCVA improved significantly from 0.21 ± 0.45 to 0.058 ± 0.38 in Group 2

(p = 0.0016). The mean BCVA did not differ significantly between the two groups at baseline and 5–7 months postoperatively. The mean surgical times for Groups 1 and 2 were 17.3 ± 5.7 min and 20.9 ± 6.9 min, respectively.

Table 1. Patient characteristics.

	Group 1	Group 2	p
Number of Eyes	20	20	
Mean age (range), years	72.7 ± 9.4 (51–85)	74.2 ± 6.5 (60–82)	0.73
Sex			
Male	9 (45.0%)	5 (25.0%)	
Female	11 (55.0%)	15 (75.0%)	
Eye			
Right	7 (35.0%)	8 (40.0%)	
Left	13 (65.0%)	12 (60.0%)	
Glaucoma Type			
POAG	9 (45.0%)	9 (45.0%)	
EXG	3 (15.0%)	6 (30.0%)	
SIG	3 (15.0%)	2 (10.0%)	
UG	3 (15.0%)	2 (10.0%)	
Other	2 (10.0%)	1 (5.0%)	
Visual field mean deviation (dB)	−7.6 ± 6.4	−7.2 ± 7.3	0.57
Follow-up (months)	6.0 ± 0.73	5.6 ± 0.75	0.13

POAG, primary open angle glaucoma. EXG, exfoliation glaucoma. SIG, steroid induced glaucoma. UG, uveitis glaucoma.

Table 2. Surgical results.

	Group 1	Group 2	p
IOP (mmHg)			
Preoperative	26.1 ± 12.3	20.6 ± 8.8	0.13
Postoperative	14.1 ± 3.3	12.9 ± 3.2	0.33
Medication			
Preoperative	4.0 (3–5)	3.5 (2–4.25)	0.11
Postoperative	2.5 (2–3)	1.0 (0–3)	0.06
BCVA (logMAR)			
Preoperative	0.28 ± 0.28	0.21 ± 0.45	0.13
Postoperative	−0.040 ± 0.18	0.058 ± 0.38	0.55
Surgical time (min)	17.3 ± 5.7	20.9 ± 6.9	0.13

IOP, intraocular pressure; BCVA, best-corrected visual acuity; MAR, the minimum angle of resolution.

Figure 2 shows the Kaplan–Meier survival curves used to compare the surgical outcomes between Groups 1 and 2. The success rates in Groups 1 and 2 were 53.3% and 65.0%, respectively (p = 0.54).

Table 3 lists the complications and subsequent interventions. All cases showed intraoperative blood reflux into the anterior chamber from the incised angle. Postoperative hyphema with niveau formation in Groups 1 and 2 was observed in one eye and six eyes, respectively. In five of these eyes, the hyphema resolved spontaneously within 1 week postoperatively without any intervention. However, we performed hyphema washout about a week after the surgery in two eyes of Group 2 that showed no tendency to improve. The patients who had taken any anticoagulants were two of Group 2, but they did not show postoperative hyphema with niveau formation. Postoperative transient IOP elevation was observed in three eyes in Group 1 and four eyes in Group 2, all of which normalized within 1 week following the administration of glaucoma medications. Postoperative blood accumulation in the lens bag was observed in one eye in Group 2, which was treated with Nd:YAG laser capsulotomy to spread the accumulated blood.

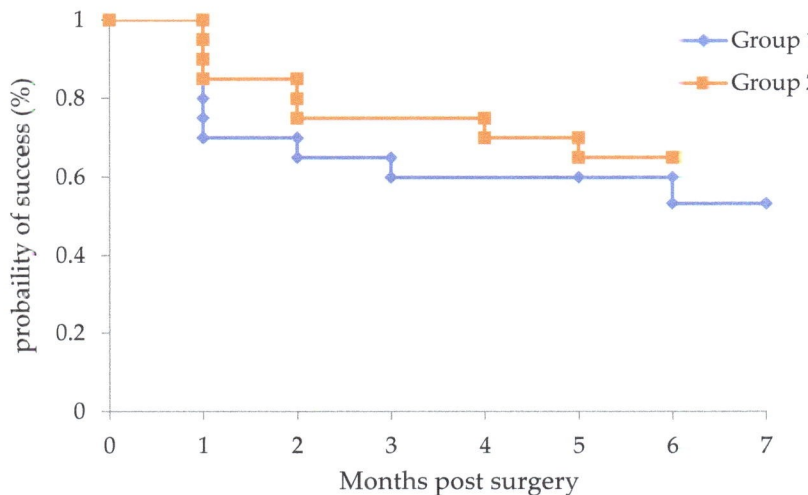

Figure 2. Kaplan–Meier survival curves showing the success rate of IOP control after surgery. Surgical success was defined as: (1) 6 ≤ IOP ≤ 21, and a reduction by more than 20% with or without antiglaucoma medications; (2) no loss of light perception; (3) no additional glaucoma surgery. Transient IOP elevation within 1 month postoperatively was considered an IOP spike and not classified as surgical failure.

Table 3. Complications and interventions.

	Group 1	Group 2	p
Intraoperative complications			
Blood reflux	20 (100%)	20 (100%)	
Postoperative complications			
Hyphema with niveau formation	1 (5.0%)	6 (30.0%)	0.046
Transient IOP elevation (>30 mmHg)	3 (15.0%)	4 (20.0%)	0.50
Blood accumulation in the lens bag	0	1 (5.0%)	0.50
Postoperative intervention			
Hyphema washout	0	2 (10.0%)	0.24
Nd:YAG laser capsulotomy	0	1 (5.0%)	0.50

4. Discussion

Generally, trabeculectomy remains the gold standard of glaucoma surgery that can significantly reduce IOP. However, trabeculectomy can result in severe postoperative complications, such as hypotony maculopathy, choroidal hemorrhage, bleb infections, and endophthalmitis. In contrast, LOT is less likely to induce postoperative vision-threatening complications after trabeculectomy, but postoperative hyphema is likely to occur [1,14].

In our study, all cases showed intraoperative blood reflux from the incised angle into the anterior chamber. This intraoperative hemorrhage is common in μLCT and other MIGS procedures [12,15,16]. Blood reflux occurs when unroofing Schlemm's canal in the setting of intraoperative hypotony and should be considered an expected event in these surgical procedures. The incidence of postoperative hyphema with niveau formation in Group 2 was 30.0%, which was similar to that reported in a previous study of combined cataract surgery and μLOT [12]. In a previous study of μLOT only [15], postoperative hyphema with niveau formation occurred in 38% of cases, a rate similar to those in a previous study [12] and to that of Group 2 in the present study. Gonioscopy-assisted transluminal trabeculotomy (GATT) is another ab interno trabeculotomy similar to μLOT [17,18]. The common postoperative complication of GATT is hyphema, and the rate of hyphema is reportedly approximately

30% [19,20]. Hyphema is the most common postoperative complication of all types of LOT. A recent study has also revealed that 31% of 560 eyes that underwent μLOT alone or μLOT combined with cataract surgery had hyphema with niveau formation [11]. However, the incidence of postoperative hyphema with niveau formation in Group 1 was 5.0%, significantly lower than the incidence in Group 2. This is because perfusion pressure during cataract surgery may help prevent postoperative hyphema. In Group 1, perfusion pressure during cataract surgery after μLOT increased the intraoperative IOP and compressed the incised wound. As a result, intraoperative blood reflux was reduced, and postoperative hyphema was less likely to occur. In contrast, in Group 2 and previous studies [12,15], μLOT was performed after or without cataract surgery. Therefore, a reduction in intraoperative blood reflux due to perfusion pressure could not be expected. That is, to avoid postoperative hyphema with niveau formation, μLOT should be performed before rather than after cataract surgery when μLOT and cataract surgery are combined.

The procedures in Groups 1 and 2 have advantages. The advantages of performing μLOT before cataract surgery include obtaining a good gonioscopic view through a clear cornea and avoiding anterior chamber instability from the large keratome incision used in cataract surgery. In contrast, the advantages of performing μLOT after cataract surgery include obtaining good visibility of the trabecular meshwork in the open angle due to cataract removal. However, regardless of the procedure used, μLOT combined with cataract surgery was completed successfully in our study because the ease of performing this surgery was not affected. We observed no significant difference in surgical times between Groups 1 and 2 ($p = 0.13$). The IOP and number of antiglaucoma medications preoperatively and 5–7 months postoperatively did not differ significantly between Groups 1 and 2. Tanito et al. reported that μLOT combined with cataract surgery decreased the mean IOP and number of antiglaucoma medications from 16.4 mmHg and 2.4 preoperatively to 11.8 mmHg and 2.1 at the final 9.5-month evaluation [12], similar to the outcomes in Groups 1 and 2 in the present study.

The limitations of our study are the small sample size, the non-randomized nature of the study, and the short follow-up period. To clarify the differences in clinical outcomes of μLOT before and after cataract surgery, a larger number of cases and longer follow-up periods are needed. Furthermore, randomized studies should be performed to eliminate biases such as patient backgrounds.

In conclusion, the results of our study showed that both μLOT before and after cataract surgery effectively reduced the IOP and number of antiglaucoma medications. However, the incidence of postoperative hyphema with niveau formation was lower for μLOT before rather than after cataract surgery. Thus, μLOT may be better performed before cataract surgery when performing combined μLOT and cataract surgery.

Author Contributions: Conceptualization, Y.M. and K.F.; Data curation, Y.M.; Investigation, Y.M.; writing—original draft preparation, Y.M.; Supervision, K.F.; writing—review and editing, K.F. All authors have read and agreed to the published version of the manuscript.

Funding: This research received no external funding.

Institutional Review Board Statement: This retrospective study adhered to the tenets of the Declaration of Helsinki and was approved by the institutional ethics committee, which waived the requirement for informed consent as the analyzed data were de-identified.

Informed Consent Statement: Not applicable.

Data Availability Statement: Not applicable.

Conflicts of Interest: The authors declare no conflict of interest.

References

1. Chihara, E.; Nishida, A.; Kodo, M.; Yoshimura, N.; Matsumura, M.; Yamamoto, M.; Tsukada, T. Trabeculotomy ab externo: An alternative treatment in adult patients with primary open-angle glaucoma. *Ophthalmic Surg.* **1993**, *24*, 735–739. [CrossRef]
2. Tanihara, H.; Negi, A.; Akimoto, M.; Terauchi, H.; Okudaira, A.; Kozaki, J.; Takeuchi, A.; Nagata, M. Surgical effects of trabeculotomy ab externo on adult eyes with primary open angle glaucoma and pseudoexfoliation syndrome. *Arch. Ophthalmol.* **1993**, *111*, 1653–1661. [CrossRef] [PubMed]
3. Tanito, M.; Ohira, A.; Chihara, E. Surgical outcome of combined trabeculotomy and cataract surgery. *J. Glaucoma* **2001**, *10*, 302–308. [CrossRef] [PubMed]
4. Tanito, M.; Ohira, A.; Chihara, E. Factors leading to reduced intraocular pressure after combined trabeculotomy and cataract surgery. *J. Glaucoma* **2002**, *11*, 3–9. [CrossRef]
5. Francis, B.A.; Singh, K.; Lin, S.C.; Hodapp, E.; Jampel, H.D.; Samples, J.R.; Smith, S.D. Novel glaucoma procedures: A report by the American Academy of Ophthalmology. *Ophthalmology* **2011**, *118*, 1466–1480. [CrossRef]
6. Grover, D.S.; Godfrey, D.G.; Smith, O.; Feuer, W.J.; Montes de Oca, I.; Fellman, R.L. Gonioscopy-assisted transluminal trabeculotomy, ab interno trabeculotomy: Technique report and preliminary results. *Ophthalmology* **2014**, *121*, 855–861. [CrossRef]
7. Sato, T.; Hirata, A.; Mizoguchi, T. Outcomes of 360 degrees suture trabeculotomy with deep sclerectomy combined with cataract surgery for primary open angle glaucoma and coexisting cataract. *Clin. Ophthalmol.* **2014**, *8*, 1301–1310. [CrossRef]
8. Sato, T.; Hirata, A.; Mizoguchi, T. Prospective, noncomparative, nonrandomized case study of short-term outcomes of 360 degrees suture trabeculotomy ab interno in patients with open-angle glaucoma. *Clin. Ophthalmol.* **2015**, *9*, 63–68. [CrossRef]
9. Saheb, H.; Ahmed, I.I. Micro-invasive glaucoma surgery: Current perspectives and future directions. *Curr. Opin. Ophthalmol.* **2012**, *23*, 96–104. [CrossRef]
10. Tanito, M. Microhook ab interno trabeculotomy, a novel minimally invasive glaucoma surgery. *Clin. Ophthalmol.* **2018**, *12*, 43–48. [CrossRef] [PubMed]
11. Tanito, M.; Sugihara, K.; Tsutsui, A.; Hara, K.; Manabe, K.; Matsuoka, Y. Midterm results of microhook ab interno trabeculotomy in initial 560 eyes with glaucoma. *J. Clin. Med.* **2021**, *10*, 814. [CrossRef]
12. Tanito, M.; Ikeda, Y.; Fujihara, E. Effectiveness and safety of combined cataract surgery and microhook ab interno trabeculotomy in Japanese eyes with glaucoma: Report of an initial case series. *Jpn. J. Ophthalmol.* **2017**, *61*, 457–464. [CrossRef] [PubMed]
13. Hirabayashi, M.T.; King, J.T.; Lee, D.; An, J.A. Outcome of phacoemulsification combined with excisional goniotomy using the Kahook Dual Blade in severe glaucoma patients at 6 months. *Clin. Ophthalmol.* **2019**, *13*, 715–721. [CrossRef] [PubMed]
14. Kashiwagi, K.; Kogure, S.; Mabuchi, F.; Chiba, T.; Yamamoto, T.; Kuwayama, Y.; Araie, M. Change in visual acuity and associated risk factors after trabeculectomy with adjunctive mitomycin C. *Acta Ophthalmol.* **2016**, *94*, e561–e570. [CrossRef] [PubMed]
15. Tanito, M.; Sano, I.; Ikeda, Y.; Fujihara, E. Short-term results of microhook ab interno trabeculotomy, a novel minimally invasive glaucoma surgery in Japanese eyes: Initial case series. *Acta Ophthalmol.* **2017**, *95*, e354–e360. [CrossRef] [PubMed]
16. Richter, G.M.; Coleman, A.L. Minimally invasive glaucoma surgery: Current status and future prospects. *Clin. Ophthalmol.* **2016**, *10*, 189–206.
17. Fontana, L.; De Maria, M. Letter to the Editor: Surgical Management of Pseudoexfoliative Glaucoma: A Review of Current Clinical Considerations and Surgical Outcomes. *J. Glaucoma* **2021**, *30*, e378. [CrossRef] [PubMed]
18. Fontana, L.; De Maria, M.; Iannetta, D.; Moramarco, A. Gonioscopy-assisted transluminal trabeculotomy for chronic angle-closure glaucoma: Preliminary results. *Graefes Arch. Clin. Exp. Ophthalmol.* **2021**, 1–7. [CrossRef] [PubMed]
19. Grover, D.S.; Smith, O.; Fellman, R.L.; Godfrey, D.G.; Gupta, A.; de Oca, I.M.; Feuer, W.J. J. Gonioscopy assisted transluminal trabeculotomy: An ab interno circumferential trabeculotomy: 24 months follow-up. *J. Glaucoma* **2018**, *27*, 393–401. [CrossRef] [PubMed]
20. Boese, E.A.; Shah, M. Gonioscopy-assisted Transluminal Trabeculotomy (GATT) is An Effective Procedure for Steroid-induced Glaucoma. *J. Glaucoma* **2019**, *28*, 803–807. [CrossRef] [PubMed]

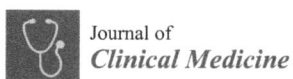 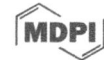

Article

Microcatheter–Assisted Circumferential Trabeculotomy in Primary Congenital Glaucoma: Long-Term Clinical Outcomes

Luigi Fontana [1,2,*] and Alberto Neri [2]

1. Ophthalmology Unit, DIMES, Alma Mater Studiorum, Ophthalmology Department, University of Bologna and S. Orsola-Malpighi Teaching Hospital, 40138 Bologna, Italy
2. Ophthalmology Unit, Azienda USL—IRCCS di Reggio Emilia, 42122 Reggio Emilia, Italy; neri.mail2@gmail.com
* Correspondence: luifonta@gmail.com

Abstract: AbstractPurpose: The purpose of this study was to report the long-term efficacy and clinical outcomes of microcatheter-assisted circumferential trabeculotomy (MCT) in children with primary congenital glaucoma (PCG). Methods: This is a single-center retrospective study including consecutive children with PCG who underwent MCT with > two years follow up. The primary outcome was surgical success, defined as intraocular pressure (IOP) ≤ 21 mmHg with (qualified) or without (complete) medications, measured at six months, one year, and then annually. Secondary outcomes were visual acuity (VA), refraction, axial length (AXL), complications, reinterventions, and number of medications. Results: Twelve eyes of ten patients were included. In eight children only one eye was affected. The mean ± standard deviation (SD) age at surgery was 6.3 ± 4.1 months. The mean postoperative follow-up was 66 ± 35 months. The mean IOP was 34.3 ± 9.6 mmHg preoperatively and 14.6 ± 2.3 mmHg postoperatively at the last visit ($p < 0.001$). Complete success was achieved at all time points in 10 out of 12 eyes, while 2 eyes had a qualified success. At three years of age, the mean VA of the operated eyes was 0.25 ± 0.12 logMAR, the mean spherical equivalent was −0.78 ± 1.43 diopters, and the mean AXL was 23.78 mm. Transient hyphema was the only complication observed. None of the children required additional glaucoma surgery. Conclusions: Circumferential trabeculotomy for PCG effectively lowers the IOP at more than two years after surgery. Following this procedure, the prognosis for the visual function is good, and the refractive error is low. Postoperative complications were not significant.

Keywords: primary congenital glaucoma; circumferential trabeculotomy; microcatheter; long-term outcomes

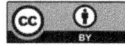

1. Introduction

Primary congenital glaucoma (PCG) is the most common non-syndromic glaucoma in childhood, occurring in one of 10,000–20,000 live births in western countries [1,2]. In PCG, the whole eye is modified and damaged by high intraocular pressure (IOP) due to isolated trabeculodysgenesis [3]. Angle surgery is the mainstay of treatment of PCG [4–6], with the choice between goniotomy and trabeculotomy dictated by corneal clarity, surgeon's experience, and preference [3,7]. The results of angle surgery are good, with most studies citing a 70% to 90% rate of success for both goniotomy and trabeculotomy [8]. However, approximately 1/3 of the iridocorneal angle is opened with both techniques, often requiring repeated procedures to obtain effective IOP control, using a step-wise approach [8]. Moreover, a metallic trabeculotome probe can create a false passage, causing tissue disruption [9].

In the attempt to improve the efficacy of angle surgery, Beck and Lynch described 360° trabeculotomy using a 6-0 prolene suture [9], modifying a technique introduced by Smith in 1960 [10]. Circumferential trabeculotomy (CTT) showed at least the same success rate of repeated goniotomy or trabeculotomy with the advantage of a single surgical procedure [11]. Lately, the availability of illuminated microcatheters has improved the safety of CTT, avoiding the potentially serious complications of suture misdirection into the suprachoroidal and subretinal space [12]. As a result, microcatheter-assisted circumferential trabeculotomy (MCT) is increasingly used worldwide as primary surgical technique in PCG. Still, the reported outcomes of this procedure are mostly limited to a short-term (12–24 months) [12–15]. Herein we report the long-term clinical outcomes of MCT for PCG in a tertiary referral center.

2. Materials and Methods

2.1. Settings

In this single-center retrospective study, we analyzed the clinical outcomes of patients with PCG treated by MCT at the Ophthalmology Unit of Azienda USL–IRCCS di Reggio Emilia (Reggio Emilia, Italy) from January 2011 to January 2021. The study was approved by the local Institutional Review Board (registration number: 170/2021/OSS/AUSLRE) for the collection of clinical data and was conducted in accordance with the principles of the Declaration of Helsinki. In addition, written informed consent was obtained from the parents of eligible children after a thorough explanation of the risk and benefits of the procedure.

2.2. Participants

Clinical data were extracted from the hospital records. Data from children with at least two years of follow-up after surgery were included for the analysis. Patients with shorter follow-up, other types of pediatric glaucoma, previous ocular surgeries, and coexisting ocular pathologies were excluded.

2.3. Data Collection

The data collected included basic demographic information, complete eye examination at baseline and at each follow-up visit, glaucoma medications, surgical procedure details, operative complications, late complications, and reinterventions. Eye examination included IOP values and measurement technique, slit lamp examination, gonioscopy and fundoscopy, refraction, visual acuity (VA) (Logarithm of the Minimum Angle of Resolution, LogMAR), and stereopsis (Lang Stereotest). In unilateral cases, clinical data of the fellow eyes were also collected.

The primary outcome was IOP measured at 6 months, 12 months, and then annually. Success was defined as postoperative IOP > 5 and ≤21 mmHg, with an IOP reduction > 20% from baseline, measured at each postoperative time point, with (qualified success) or without (complete success) glaucoma drops. Eyes were classified as failing if IOP > 21 was measured on two consecutive study visits despite maximum glaucoma therapy or if additional glaucoma surgery was performed. Secondary outcomes were complications, reinterventions, number of medications after surgery, axial length, VA (LogMAR), and refraction.

Baseline and postoperative clinical measurements were conducted by two observers (AN, LF). During examination under anesthesia (EUA), IOP was measured in the early phase of anesthesia (sevoflurane induction before intubation using a hand-held Perkins applanation tonometer (Perkins Tonomter MK2; Clement Clark Ophthalmic, Harlow, UK) or a hand-held rebound tonometer (ICare Pro, Icare Finland OY, Helsinki, Finland) in case of corneal edema precluding applanation tonometry. In addition, a-scan axial length measurements were conducted at each EUA visit (Compact Touch, Quentel Medical, France).

2.4. Surgical Technique

All of the surgical procedures were performed by a single clinician (LF) under general anesthesia. The surgical technique used was similar to the one described by Sarkisian et al. [12], using a temporal approach (Figure 1). First, a limbal stay suture was applied using a spatulated 6-0 vicryl. After a temporal conjunctival peritomy, a limbus-based superficial scleral flap of 4 × 4 mm was fashioned using a crescent blade. Then, a radial cut in the deep sclera was performed with a slit knife, posteriorly to the limbus, and progressively deepened until aqueous percolation was observed. Schlemm's canal (SC) was identified by introducing a 5.0 prolene suture cauterized at the tip. Prolene suture was then removed, and an illuminated microcatheter (iTrack 250A; iScience Interventional, Menlo Park, CA) was threaded into the SC and gently advanced along the canal circumferentially for 360°.

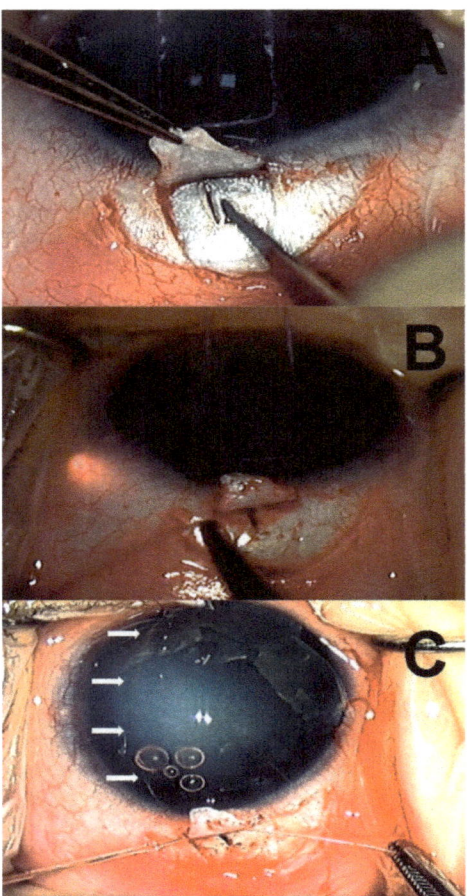

Figure 1. Surgical technique. (**A**) Following conjunctival peritomy, a limbus-based scleral flap is fashioned, then a radial cut in the deep sclera is performed with a slit knife, posteriorly to the limbus, and progressively deepened until the outer wall of the Schlemm canal (SC) is cut. (**B**) An illuminated microcatheter (iTrack 250A; iScience Interventional, Menlo Park, CA, USA) is advanced along the canal circumferentially for 360°. (**C**) Once circumnavigation of the SC is accomplished, both ends of the microcatheter are pulled, creating a 360° internal opening of the SC and trabecular meshwork.

In cases where the microcatheter tip met with an obstruction within SC or became misdirected, catheterization was attempted in the opposite direction, and viscoelastic was injected through the microcatheter in attempt to dilate the canal. If SC could not be identified, catheterization was tried at a different quadrant (supero-temporal or infero-temporal). Once circumnavigation of the SC was accomplished, the anterior chamber was deepened by injecting dispersive viscoelastic (Eyefill, Bausch and Lomb, Bridgewater, NJ,

USA), and both ends of the microcatheter were pulled, creating a 360° internal opening of the SC and TM. Finally, the catheter was removed, and the scleral flap was secured using a 10-0 vicryl suture to prevent the creation of a filtering bleb.

After surgery, topical therapy included pilocarpine 10 mg/dL eye drops TID for three weeks, dexamethasone 0.1% and tobramycin 0.3% eye drops combined, administered every three hours during the first week and then tapered progressively during the following three weeks according to the surgeon's discretion. Patients were seen on days 1, 7 and 14 after surgery to observe the anterior chamber for shallowing and hyphema. EUAs were performed at one month, three months, six months, and yearly thereafter.

2.5. Statistical Analysis

Statistical analysis was performed with Microsoft Excel v. 16.42 (Microsoft Corporation, Redmond, WA, USA) and Statplus:mac v. 8 (AnalystSoft, Walnut, CA, USA). Kolmogorov-Smirnov Test (with Lilliefors correction) was used to assess if data had a normal distribution. Then, for data with normal distribution, paired t-test was used to compare repeated measurements of the same eyes, and independent t-test was used to compare affected and unaffected eyes. The Mann-Whitney test was used for data without normal distribution. Kaplan-Meyer survival analysis was performed to analyze the surgical success. Finally, power analysis of results was performed post-hoc using confidence intervals for binomi.

3. Results

The records of 14 children with PCG who underwent MCT during the study period were retrieved. Two patients with bilateral glaucoma and cataracts and two patients with follow-up <2 years were excluded. Twelve eyes of ten patients met the inclusion/exclusion criteria mentioned above. In eight children only one eye was affected. The mean age at surgery was 6.2 ± 4.2 months (3.5 ± 0.83 months and 9.0 ± 4.3 months for male and female, respectively), and mean follow-up was 66 ± 35 months (range 24–121 months). All of the children underwent surgery within two weeks of diagnosis.

Characteristics of the patients included into the study are resumed in Table 1. At the time of surgery, mean IOP, axial length, and corneal diameter were 36.33 ± 9.63 mmHg, 22.67 ± 0.67 mm and 13.25 ± 0.39 mm in the affected eyes, and 13.25 ± 4.92 mmHg, 19.62 ± 1.01 mm and 11.75 ± 0.46 mm, in the not affected eyes ($p < 0.001$ for all comparisons). All of the eyes with PCG had corneal edema at the time of surgery, and 8 out of 12 eyes presented Haab striae. Four eyes received treatment with glaucoma drops before surgery (pilocarpine 1% combined with dorzolamide or betaxolol). Glaucoma medications were suspended after surgery in all patients.

Table 1. Characteristics of the study population.

Patient	Sex	Ethnicity	Eye	Age at Surgery (Months)	Pre-Op. IOP (mmHG)	Pre-Op. AXL (mm)	Haab Striae	Degrees of Trab.	Intraop. Events	IOP (Months of F.U.) (mmHg)	Glaucoma Drugs
1	F	Caucasian	R	7	30	22.45	Yes	360°	-	14 (104)	No
2	M	Hispanic	R	4	35	23.00	Yes	360°	2nd scleral incision	14 (55)	No
			L	5	30	22.00	No	360°	-	14 (55)	No
3	F	Caucasian	L	6	28	22.14	Yes	360°	Viscoelastic inj.	17 (52)	No
4	F	Caucasian	L	17	58	23.90	No	360°	-	18 (46)	Brinzolamide and travoprost
5	M	Pakistani	L	3	30	22.38	Yes	360°	2nd scleral incision	11 (26)	No

Table 1. Cont.

Patient	Sex	Ethnicity	Eye	Age at Surgery (Months)	Pre-Op. IOP (mmHG)	Pre-Op. AXL (mm)	Haab Striae	Degrees of Trab.	Intraop. Events	IOP (Months of F.U.) (mmHg)	Glaucoma Drugs
6	F	Caucasian	R	7	30	22.05	Yes	360°	-	14 (100)	No
7	F	Caucasian	L	6	28	22.10	Yes	360°	-	14 (47)	No
8	M	Caucasian	R	3	35	22.90	Yes	360°	-	16 (121)	No
			L	3	28	23.22	Yes	360°	2nd scleral incision	16 (121)	No
9	F	Caucasian	L	11	50	23.75	No	360°	Viscoelastic inj.	17 (49)	Tafluprost
10	M	Indian	R	3	30	22.18	Yes	360°	-	11 (24)	No

Pre-op = Pre-operative; Trab = trabeculotomy extension; Intraop = intraoperative; Inj = injection; IOP = intraocular pressure; F.U. = follow up.

A complete 360° trabeculotomy was achieved in all eyes. In three cases, a second scleral incision in the infero-temporal quadrant was required to locate the SC, and in two cases, catheter reinsertion and viscoelastic injection were required to complete canalization. Immediately after surgery, a moderate hyphema was observed in all patients that spontaneously resolved within two weeks. In three cases, transient shallowing of the anterior chamber was noted one week after surgery, while other postoperative complications were not encountered.

In 10 out of 12 eyes, complete success was achieved during the study period, while two eyes had a qualified success, one (case 4) requiring two glaucoma medications (brinzolamide and travoprost), and one (case 9) a single drug (tafluprost). No cases of failure occurred during the time encompassed by this study (alpha = 0.05, CI 93.98–100%). Kaplan–Meier curves for complete and qualified success are shown in Figure 2.

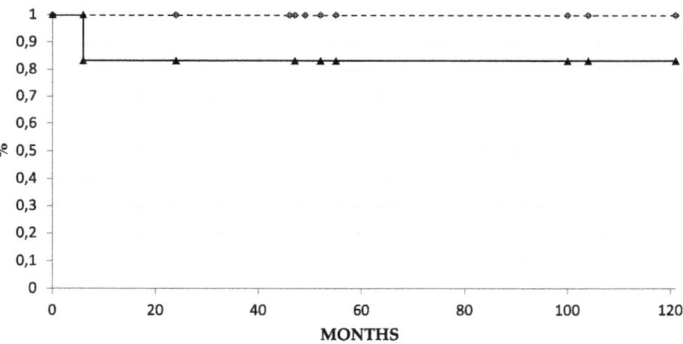

Figure 2. Kaplan-Meier survival analysis for surgical success. Solid line represents complete success (IOP ≤ 21 mmHg without glaucoma medications), dashed line represents qualified success (IOP ≤ 21 mmHg with or without glaucoma medications). Diamonds and triangles represent single patients at their last follow up visit.

Mean postoperative IOP was 14.2 ± 4.1 mmHg at six months, 14.8 ± 3.2 mmHg at one year, 13.7 ± 3.9 mmHg at two years, 14.64 ± 3.7 mmHg at three years, 15.3 ± 1.9 mmHg at four years, and 15.0 ± 2.4 mmHg at five years, while mean IOP of the fellow eyes was 13.5 ± 4.4 mmHg, 15.2 ± 3.0 mmHg, 14.0 ± 4.2 mmHg, 15.7 ± 2.6 mmHg, 15.0 ± 2.4 mmHg, and 14.0 ± 0.0 mmHg, at the same time points ($p > 0.5$ for all comparisons). Figures 3 and 4 show the values of preoperative and postoperative IOP through 5 years of follow-up. At the last evaluation (12 eyes, mean follow-up time 66 ± 35 months), mean postoperative IOP was 14.6 ± 2.2 mmHg, corresponding to a mean IOP lowering of 57.4% from baseline

($p < 0.001$, statistical power 100%). In the non-operated fellow eyes, the mean IOP was 14.2 ± 3.1 mmHg, unvaried from preoperative ($p > 0.5$).

In patients younger than three years, the examiners judged VA measurements unreliable due to poor child cooperation and were not included in the analysis. At three years of age, the mean VA of the operated eyes was 0.25 ± 0.12 logMAR (10 eyes). In unilateral patients (six eyes), mean VA was 0.26 ± 0.12 logMAR and 0.00 ± 0.00 logMAR, in the operated and fellow eyes, respectively ($p < 0.001$). Amblyopia, when present (seven eyes), was treated with spectacles prescription and patching.

Refraction at three years showed a mean spherical equivalent (SE) of -1.06 ± 1.59 and $+0.62 \pm 1.48$ diopters (D), and mean astigmatism of 1.37 ± 1.43 and 0.50 ± 0.65 D, in the affected and fellow eyes, respectively ($p < 0.05$ for all comparisons). At last evaluation (12 eyes, mean follow-up time 66 ± 35 months), the mean SE and refractive cylinder were -0.96 ± 1.93 D and 0.75 ± 1.43 D in the operated eyes, and $+1.8 \pm 1.01$ D and 1.06 ± 0.77 D in fellow eyes. At the same time point, the mean axial length was 23.78 ± 0.32 mm and 21.91 ± 0.10 mm in the affected and fellow eyes, respectively ($p < 0.001$).

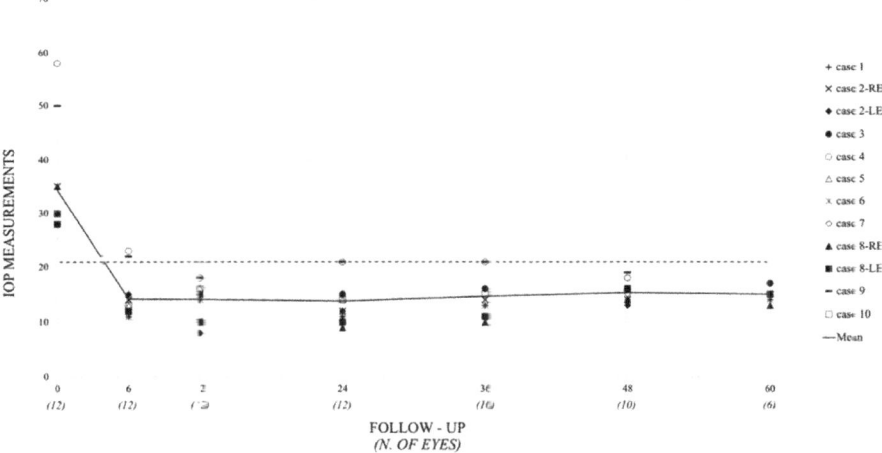

Figure 3. Scatterplot of preoperative and postoperative intraocular pressure (IOP) (mmHg) (Y axis) and follow-up (months) (X axis). The value of IOP for each patient is represented at different postoperative time intervals. The dashed line indicates the 21 mmHg IOP value. The solid line indicates the mean IOP value. For children who underwent surgery in both eyes, IOP values are represented independently (RE, right eye; LE, left eye). N = number.

Strabismus was found in 5 out of 10 patients, four with unilateral and one with bilateral PCG. Among the patients with strabismus, two had esotropia, one exotropia, and two exophoria/tropia. One patient with esotropia had strabismus surgery at six years. Stereopsis was present in 7 out of 10 patients.

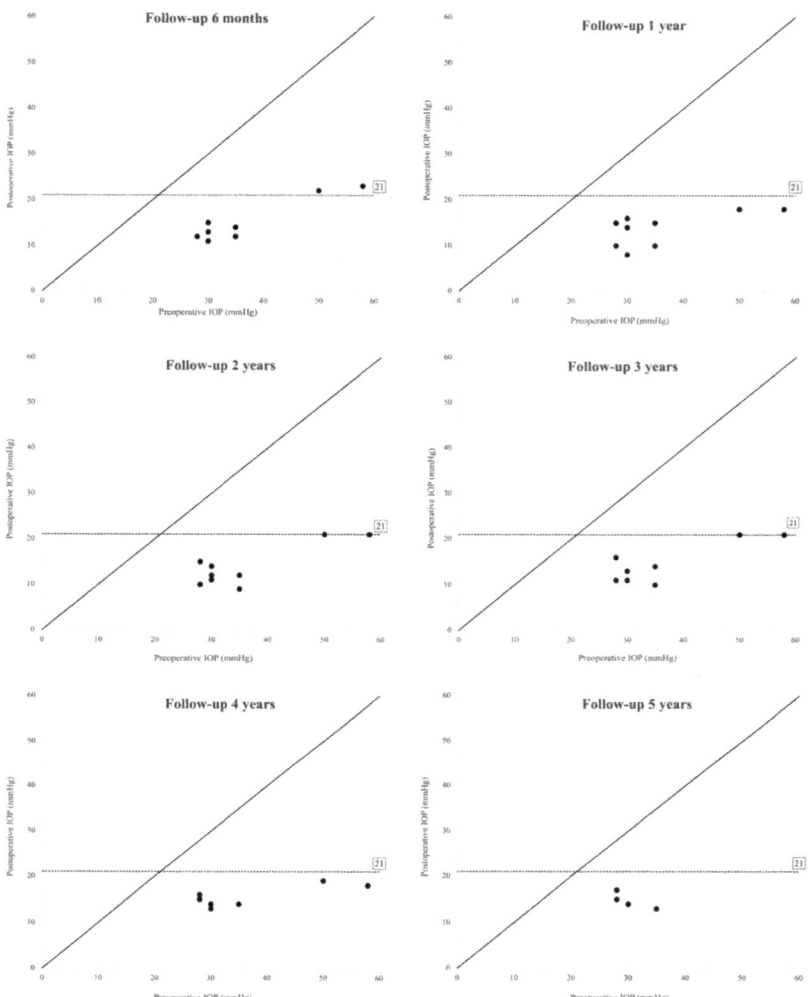

Figure 4. Scatterplot of preoperative (X axis) and postoperative (Y axis) intraocular pressure (IOP) (mmHg) at six months, one, two, three, four, and five years after surgery. The value of IOP for each operated eye is represented with a black dot. The dashed line indicates the 21 mmHg value. Equality between preoperative and postoperative measurements is represented with a solid line.

4. Discussion

PCG is a blinding condition with challenging treatment, where the first operation chosen is often the best chance of long-term success for the patient [4–7].

The current study found that MCT successfully lowered the IOP in PCG patients at more than two years after surgery. The majority of our patients (10 out of 12 eyes) met and maintained the criteria of success defined in this study through the follow-up without the use of glaucoma medications, and none required additional glaucoma surgery. After MCT, an average IOP in the mid-teens was recorded at six months and one, two, three, four, and five years, and at last follow-up visit, corresponding to an IOP lowering of >30% from baseline. Previous studies comparing the results of MCT to conventional angle surgery (goniotomy and segmental trabeculotomy) reported high rates of medication-free postoperative success after MCT in the short term [14–17] and in the long-term [11,18], suggesting that a single 360° trabeculotomy may be at least equally or more effective than repeated conventional angle surgery procedures [14–17,19]. Multiple surgical procedures increase the risk of surgery-related complications (i.e., iris damage and cataract) and expose the children to the consequences of repeated general anesthesia [20]. A recent metanalysis by Ling et al. confirmed that, compared with conventional trabeculotomy, MCT resulted in better IOP control, higher success rate, and fewer medications in the early postoperative follow-up period (3 to 12 months) [21]. In a large number of pediatric glaucoma cases, encompassing various diagnoses, Berger et al. reported a higher IOP reduction at one year after MCT compared to conventional angle surgery by goniotomy and trabeculotomy [16]. In this study, the percentage of IOP reduction at one year was 52%, similar to one reported in our study (58%) at the same time point, and in other studies reporting the short term IOP reduction (6 to 24 months) after MCT: El Sayed and Gawdat (54%) [14], Sarkisian et al. (57%) [12], Temkar et al. (49%) [17], and Girkin et al. (52%) [13].

Several factors may explain the high percentage of SC cannulation and IOP lowering success rate reported in our study. First, our analysis was focused on a homogeneous population of children with isolated trabeculodysgenesis. Second, most of the patients included presented unilateral PCG with age at surgery of more than six months, possibly suggesting the presence of less abnormal anatomy of the SC than the one found in children presenting glaucoma at birth. Finally, all surgical procedures were conducted by a single surgeon experienced with ab-externo canaloplasty.

Trabeculotomy for PCG has witnessed a progressive evolution from segmental to circumferential incision, from the employment of metal instruments to modified monofilament sutures, and finally, dedicated microcatheter. During the last decade, MCT has been proposed as the procedure of choice for childhood glaucoma as it is associated with a higher success rate, lower IOP, reduced medication use, low risk of complications, and more favorable visual outcome compared to traditional angle surgery by goniotomy or segmental trabeculotomy [16,18]. Following MCT, the reported IOP lowering success rates varies from 49 to 92%, according to the different criteria adopted to define success in the various studies [14–17,19], whereas, after segmental trabeculotomy, the probability of success after a single operation varies from 31 to 50% [11,14,16,18,19]. This difference may have a twofold explanation: with traditional trabeculotomy, using rigid Harms probe, approximately 90°–120° of the SC may be opened with a single operation, compared to the 360° canal opening that may be achieved using a suture or a catheter; secondly using a suture, and moreover, with an illuminated catheter, the surgeon may be sure to cannulate the entirety of the SC or at least an extensive length of its course, being certain of the correct anatomical position of the device, therefore reducing the risk of complications related to SC miscannulation or false passage (i.e., iris damage, cyclodialysis, lens damage, sub-retinal misdirection) [9,22]. In our series, complete cannulation of SC was achieved in all treated eyes with only a few complications observed: transient hyphema and anterior chamber shallowing. Similarly, sporadic cases of severe complications are reported in the literature after MCT (i.e., cataract, endophthalmitis) [14]. It is noteworthy that none of the patients in our study developed lens opacities after surgery.

There is evidence of greater IOP lowering after complete circumferential trabeculotomy than partial (180° or more) trabeculotomy [12,15,23]. Using an illuminated microcatheter, the percentage of complete trabeculotomy varies according to the surgeon's experience and the treated cases' selection. In the early description of the MCT technique, Sarkisian achieved complete 360° trabeculotomy in 75% of the PCG patients treated [12], similar percentages with the same technique were reported by Temkar et al. (80%) [17], Berger at al. (80%) [16], Shakrawal et al. (80%) [15], and less frequently by Girkin et al. (25%) [19] and Rojas et al. (21%) [23]. Likewise, a high percentage of circumferential trabeculotomy may be achieved using a monofilament suture [11]. The relevance of achieving an extensive trabecular and SC opening at first surgery may recommend using an illuminated-microcatheter rather than a monofilament suture to facilitate and improve the accuracy of this procedure.

However, no comparative analysis of the rate of SC cannulation using both devices is currently available. Furthermore, using the temporal approach adopted in this study, the superior bulbar conjunctiva and sclera are spared for future filtering surgery should it be required for IOP control.

Surgical advances in the treatment of pediatric glaucoma reflect the improvement in the visual outcomes reported in several studies investigating the visual prognosis in these children. A useful visual acuity (>20/200) may be achieved in the majority of the eyes affected by various pediatric glaucoma subtypes [24]. Children with PCG are reported to have a better visual prognosis than those affected by secondary forms of glaucoma, with 70% of the eyes achieving a VA > 20/70 [24]. Similarly, in our study, eyes with PCG showed a mean VA of 0.25 logMAR (20/32) at the last follow-up visit with low refractive error and surgery-induced astigmatism. Due to the frequency of unilateral cases in our study, management of amblyopia was required in the majority of patients.

Interestingly, following the IOP reduction achieved after surgery, we observed an equal increment of the AXL with time in the operated eyes and fellow eyes of children with unilateral PCG. Furthermore, during the length of time encompassed by our study, none of the patients with unilateral PCG developed elevated IOP in the non-affected eye.

The strength of our study is the homogeneity of the childhood glaucoma cases included in the analysis and the longer follow-up time than many of the published reports. Limitations are the retrospective nature, common to most studies, small number of patients and lack of a control population.

In conclusion, our study shows that MCT is highly effective and safe in PCG, providing IOP control and stability at more than two years after surgery without the need for further glaucoma surgery, with absence of significant complications, and good visual outcomes.

Author Contributions: Data curation, A.N.; Investigation, L.F. and A.N.; Project administration, L.F.; Writing—original draft, L.F. and A.N. All authors have read and agreed to the published version of the manuscript.

Funding: This research received no external funding.

Institutional Review Board Statement: The study was conducted according to the guidelines of the Declaration of Helsinki, and approved by the Ethics Committee of AUSL Reggio Emilia (registration number: 170/2021/OSS/AUSLRE).

Informed Consent Statement: Informed consent was obtained from all subjects involved in the study.

Data Availability Statement: Data may be made available upon request.

Conflicts of Interest: The authors declare no conflict of interest.

References

1. Taylor, R.H.; Ainsworth, J.R.; Evans, A.R.; Levin, A.V. The Epidemiology of Pediatric Glaucoma: The Toronto Experience. *J. Am. Assoc. Pediatric Ophthalmol. Strabismus* **1999**, *3*, 308–315. [CrossRef]
2. Papadopoulos, M.; Cable, N.; Rahi, J.; Khaw, P.T.; BIG Eye Study Investigators. The British Infantile and Childhood Glaucoma (BIG) Eye Study. *Investig. Ophthalmol. Vis. Sci.* **2007**, *48*, 4100–4106. [CrossRef]
3. Chang, T.C.P.; Brookes, J.; Cavuoto, K.; Bitrian, E.; Alana, L. Grajewski Primary Congenital Glaucoma and Juvenile Open-Angle Glaucoma. In *Childhood Glaucoma*; WGA Consensus Series; Weinreb, R.N., Grajewski, A., Papadopoulos, M., Grigg, J., Freedman, S., Eds.; Kugler Publications: Amsterdam, The Netherlands, 2013.
4. Inaba, Z. Long-Term Results of Trabeculectomy in the Japanese: An Analysis by Life-Table Method. *Jpn. J. Ophthalmol.* **1982**, *26*, 361–373.
5. Broadway, D.C.; Grierson, I.; Hitchings, R.A. Local Effects of Previous Conjunctival Incisional Surgery and the Subsequent Outcome of Filtration Surgery. *Am. J. Ophthalmol.* **1998**, *125*, 805–818. [CrossRef]
6. Dietlein, T.S.; Jacobi, P.C.; Krieglstein, G.K. Prognosis of Primary Ab Externo Surgery for Primary Congenital Glaucoma. *Br. J. Ophthalmol.* **1999**, *83*, 317–322. [CrossRef]
7. Khaw, P.T.; Freedman, S.; Gandolfi, S. Management of Congenital Glaucoma. *J. Glaucoma* **1999**, *8*, 81–85. [CrossRef] [PubMed]
8. Papadopoulos, M.; Edmunds, B.; Fenerty, C.; Khaw, P.T. Childhood Glaucoma Surgery in the 21st Century. *Eye* **2014**, *28*, 931–943. [CrossRef]

9. Beck, A.D.; Lynch, M.G. 360 Degrees Trabeculotomy for Primary Congenital Glaucoma. *Arch. Ophthalmol.* **1995**, *113*, 1200–1202. [CrossRef] [PubMed]
10. Smith, R. A New Technique for Opening the Canal of Schlemm. Preliminary Report. *Br. J. Ophthalmol.* **1960**, *44*, 370–373. [CrossRef] [PubMed]
11. Mendicino, M.E.; Lynch, M.G.; Drack, A.; Beck, A.D.; Harbin, T.; Pollard, Z.; Vela, M.A.; Lynn, M.J. Long-Term Surgical and Visual Outcomes in Primary Congenital Glaucoma: 360° Trabeculotomy versus Goniotomy. *J. Am. Assoc. Pediatric Ophthalmol. Strabismus* **2000**, *4*, 205–210. [CrossRef] [PubMed]
12. Sarkisian, S.R. An Illuminated Microcatheter for 360-Degree Trabeculectomy in Congenital Glaucoma: A Retrospective Case Series. *J. Am. Assoc. Pediatric Ophthalmol. Strabismus* **2010**, *14*, 412–416. [CrossRef] [PubMed]
13. Girkin, C.A.; Marchase, N.; Cogen, M.S. Circumferential Trabeculotomy with an Illuminated Microcatheter in Congenital Glaucomas. *J. Glaucoma* **2012**, *21*, 160–163. [CrossRef] [PubMed]
14. El Sayed, Y.; Gawdat, G. Two-Year Results of Microcatheter-Assisted Trabeculotomy in Paediatric Glaucoma: A Randomized Controlled Study. *Acta Ophthalmol.* **2017**, *95*, e713–e719. [CrossRef] [PubMed]
15. Shakrawal, J.; Bali, S.; Sidhu, T.; Verma, S.; Sihota, R.; Dada, T. Randomized Trial on Illuminated-Microcatheter Circumferential Trabeculotomy Versus Conventional Trabeculotomy in Congenital Glaucoma. *Am. J. Ophthalmol.* **2017**, *180*, 158–164. [CrossRef] [PubMed]
16. Berger, O.; Mohamed-Noriega, J.; Low, S.; Daniel, M.C.; Petchyim, S.; Papadopoulos, M.; Brookes, J. From Conventional Angle Surgery to 360-Degree Trabeculotomy in Pediatric Glaucoma. *Am. J. Ophthalmol.* **2020**, *219*, 77–86. [CrossRef]
17. Temkar, S.; Gupta, S.; Sihota, R.; Sharma, R.; Angmo, D.; Pujari, A.; Dada, T. Illuminated Microcatheter Circumferential Trabeculotomy Versus Combined Trabeculotomy-Trabeculectomy for Primary Congenital Glaucoma: A Randomized Controlled Trial. *Am. J. Ophthalmol.* **2015**, *159*, 490–497.e2. [CrossRef]
18. Neustein, R.F.; Beck, A.D. Circumferential Trabeculotomy Versus Conventional Angle Surgery: Comparing Long-Term Surgical Success and Clinical Outcomes in Children with Primary Congenital Glaucoma. *Am. J. Ophthalmol.* **2017**, *183*, 17–24. [CrossRef]
19. Girkin, C.A.; Rhodes, L.; McGwin, G.; Marchase, N.; Cogen, M.S. Goniotomy versus Circumferential Trabeculotomy with an Illuminated Microcatheter in Congenital Glaucoma. *J. Am. Assoc. Pediatric Ophthalmol. Strabismus* **2012**, *16*, 424–427. [CrossRef]
20. Cavuoto, K.M.; Rodriguez, L.I.; Tutiven, J.; Chang, T.C. General Anesthesia in the Pediatric Population. *Curr. Opin. Ophthalmol.* **2014**, *25*, 411–416. [CrossRef]
21. Ling, L.; Ji, K.; Li, P.; Hu, Z.; Xing, Y.; Yu, Y.; Zhou, W. Microcatheter-Assisted Circumferential Trabeculotomy versus Conventional Trabeculotomy for the Treatment of Childhood Glaucoma: A Meta-Analysis. *Biomed. Res. Int.* **2020**, *2020*, 3715859. [CrossRef]
22. Gloor, B.R.P. Dangers of the 360° Suture Trabeculotomy. *Ophthalmologe* **1998**, *95*, 100–103. [CrossRef] [PubMed]
23. Rojas, C.; Bohnsack, B.L. Rate of Complete Catheterization of Schlemm's Canal and Trabeculotomy Success in Primary and Secondary Childhood Glaucomas. *Am. J. Ophthalmol.* **2020**, *212*, 69–78. [CrossRef] [PubMed]
24. Khitri, M.R.; Mills, M.D.; Yirg, G.-S.; Davidson, S.L.; Quinn, G.E. Visual Acuity Outcomes in Pediatric Glaucomas. *J. Am. Assoc. Pediatric Ophthalmol. Strabismus* **2012**, *16*, 376–381. [CrossRef] [PubMed]

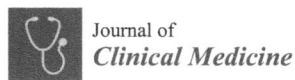

Article

Twenty-Years of Experience in Childhood Glaucoma Surgery

Felix Mathias Wagner, Alexander Karl-Georg Schuster, Franz Grehn, Lukas Urbanek, Norbert Pfeiffer, Julia Verena Stingl and Esther Maria Hoffmann *

Department of Ophthalmology, University Medical Center Mainz, Langenbeckstr. 1, 55131 Mainz, Germany; felix.wagner@unimedizin-mainz.de (F.M.W.); alexander.schuster@uni-mainz.de (A.K.-G.S.); Grehn_F@ukw.de (F.G.); l.urbanek@hotmail.com (L.U.); Norbert.Pfeiffer@unimedizin-mainz.de (N.P.); julia.stingl@unimedizin-mainz.de (J.V.S.)
* Correspondence: ehoffman@uni-mainz.de

Abstract: To quantify the results of childhood glaucoma treatment over time in a cohort of children with different types of childhood glaucoma. A retrospective cohort study of consecutive cases involving children with primary congenital glaucoma, primary juvenile, and secondary juvenile glaucoma at the Childhood Glaucoma Center, University Medical Center Mainz, Germany from 1995 to 2015 was conducted. The main outcome measure was the long-term development of intraocular pressure. Further parameters such as surgical success, refraction, corneal diameter, axial length, and surgical procedure in children with different types of childhood glaucoma were evaluated. Surgical success was defined as IOP < 21 mmHg in eyes without a need for further intervention for pressure reduction. A total of 93 glaucomatous eyes of 61 childhood glaucoma patients with a mean age of 3.7 ± 5.1 years were included. The overall mean intraocular pressure at first visit was 32.8 ± 10.2 mmHg and decreased to 15.5 ± 7.3 mmHg at the last visit. In the median follow-up time of 78.2 months, 271 surgical interventions were performed (130 of these were cyclophotocoagulations). Many (61.9%) of the eyes that underwent surgery achieved complete surgical success without additional medication. Qualified surgical success (with or without additional medication) was reached by 84.5% of the eyes.

Keywords: glaucoma; childhood glaucoma; glaucoma surgery

1. Introduction

Childhood glaucoma is a heterogeneous group of disorders that each require careful attention and understanding to prevent a lifetime of vision loss. It is characterized by intraocular pressure (IOP)-related damage to the eye and is caused by a diverse group of conditions [1,2]. The Childhood Glaucoma Research Network (CGRN) defined the following classification system for childhood glaucoma: primary glaucoma including juvenile open-angle glaucoma and primary congenital glaucoma and secondary childhood glaucoma including glaucoma following cataract surgery, glaucoma associated with nonacquired systemic disease or syndrome, glaucoma associated with nonacquired ocular anomalies, and glaucoma associated with acquired conditions [1].

Primary childhood glaucoma and secondary childhood glaucoma due to other ocular anomalies can lead to severe visual impairment and even blindness if not treated. While each of these disorders is very rare, primary congenital glaucoma (PCG) is among the most frequent [3,4]. The incidence of PCG differs between regions. In the Western world, the incidences range between 1:10,000 and 1:30,000 [3,4]. However, the incidences increase in populations with higher proportion of consanguinity [5].

Notably, the elevated IOP common to all forms of childhood glaucoma can lead to stretching of the globe's outer coats, producing corneal enlargement, scleral thinning, and axial length growth, thus leading to myopic shifts and possible anisometropia. Myopia is highly associated with childhood glaucoma and should therefore be taken into account,

Citation: Wagner, F.M.; Schuster, A.K.-G.; Grehn, F.; Urbanek, L.; Pfeiffer, N.; Stingl, J.V.; Hoffmann, E.M. Twenty-Years of Experience in Childhood Glaucoma Surgery. *J. Clin. Med.* **2021**, *10*, 5720. https://doi.org/10.3390/jcm10245720

Academic Editor: Georgios Labiris

Received: 9 October 2021
Accepted: 6 December 2021
Published: 8 December 2021

Publisher's Note: MDPI stays neutral with regard to jurisdictional claims in published maps and institutional affiliations.

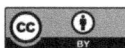

Copyright: © 2021 by the authors. Licensee MDPI, Basel, Switzerland. This article is an open access article distributed under the terms and conditions of the Creative Commons Attribution (CC BY) license (https://creativecommons.org/licenses/by/4.0/).

together with the axial length, in follow-up examinations of patients with childhood glaucoma [6]. If not treated early on, anisometropia due to a refractive change in glaucomatous eyes may lead to stimulus deprivation amblyopia, which has been reported to be one of the major causes of vision loss in these children, up to almost 50% [7].

Successful control of IOP and axial length growth is therefore crucial in the management of these conditions, along with ametropia correction and amblyopia treatment, to optimize long-term visual outcomes. Medical therapy plays a minor role in controlling IOP, except in secondary glaucoma. Surgery is the first-line treatment, especially in PCG, where angle surgery is accepted as a state-of-the-art treatment [3,8,9].

Due to its rare occurrence, there are only a few small studies and case series on the surgical treatment of childhood glaucoma. Opening of the trabecular meshwork and the Schlemm's canal is the preferred surgical approach, such as probe trabeculotomy, 360°-trabeculotomy, goniotomy, and trabeculectomy [10].

Trabeculotomy has the advantage of feasibility even with a cloudy cornea, and a 360° surgery of the angle is possible in a single procedure [11–15]. The success rates lie between 60 and 87% for the classic trabeculotomy in a follow-up period of 1–3 years [13]. The success rates of 360° trabeculotomy are between 72 and 92% in a follow-up period of 1–4 years [16]. They are particularly high if the children are operated on within the first year of life [13]. Possible complications are the presence of hyphema (although an expected result of surgery), choroidal detachment, descemetolysis, and damage of the iris or of the lens [17].

The aim of this work was to quantify the results of childhood glaucoma treatment over time, including all its different forms due to their rare occurrence. Parameters such as refraction, corneal diameter, axial length, intraocular pressure, and surgical procedure in children with different types of childhood glaucoma were evaluated at the Childhood Glaucoma Center of the University Medical Center of Mainz between the years 1995 and 2015.

2. Materials and Methods

This is a single-institution retrospective cohort study involving children with childhood glaucoma (primary congenital glaucoma (PCG), primary juvenile, and secondary juvenile glaucoma) at the Department of Ophthalmology of the University Medical Center of Mainz, from 1995 to 2015. Patients diagnosed with childhood glaucoma were included if they had glaucoma surgery between 1995 and 2015 and did not exceed the age of 18 years. Childhood glaucoma was defined according to the 9th Consensus Report of the World Glaucoma Association and further by the Childhood Glaucoma Research Network (CGRN) classification system for childhood glaucoma (Figure 1) [1,2]. Patients younger than 18 years of age, IOP > 21 mmHg, and glaucomatous optic nerve head changes without any history or signs of ocular defects were considered primary childhood glaucoma (according to the above-mentioned criteria) [1]. If ocular or systematic anomalies were responsible for elevated IOP, patients were considered to have secondary childhood glaucoma. The group with secondary childhood glaucoma was divided into glaucoma following cataract surgery (aphakic glaucoma); glaucoma associated with nonacquired systemic disease or syndrome (e.g., Sturge-Weber syndrome); glaucoma associated with nonacquired ocular anomalies (e.g., Peter's anomaly Axenfeld-Rieger syndrome, and Aniridia); and glaucoma associated with acquired conditions (e.g., trauma-induced) [2].

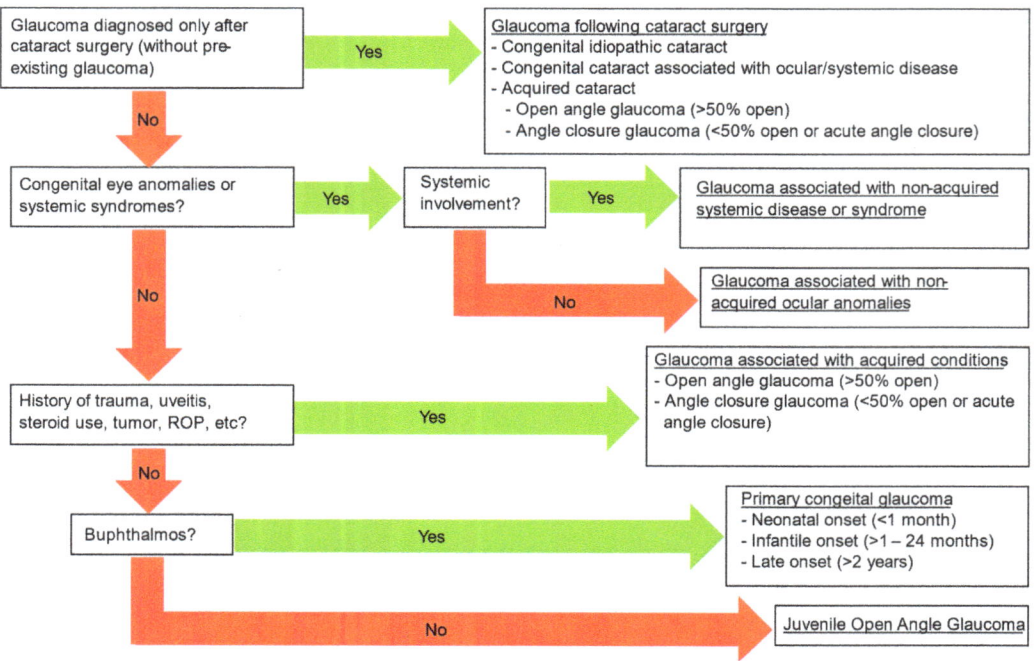

Figure 1. Childhood glaucoma categorization according to the Childhood Glaucoma Research Network classification [1].

All data were fully pseudonymized before they were analyzed. According to the regional laws, the requirement for informed consent was waived by the ethics committee of the medical board of the University Medical Center of Mainz. The study was conducted in accordance with the Declaration of Helsinki.

Patients were identified by systematic examination of the operation protocols and by searching electronic patient history data for matching ICD-10 codes (Q13 and Q15). Identified patients were screened for eligibility, and all records of suitable patients were included.

The following parameters were evaluated and documented: child's sex; birthdate; age at both glaucoma presentation and intervention; affected eye(s); all ophthalmic diagnoses; and ocular parameters such as IOP, objective refraction, corneal diameter (CD) and corneal status, optic nerve head status, and axial length (AL). The following parameters were recorded at any patient visit: glaucoma medications used (number and type), previous surgical procedures and other ophthalmic surgical procedures performed, surgical complications, IOP, anterior segment ocular features, and refractive status. The axial length, corneal diameter, central corneal thickness, IOP, and optic nerve head status were assessed under general anesthesia. IOP was measured either with Goldmann applanation tonometry (Haag-Streit AG, Koeniz, Switzerland), Perkins applanation tonometry (Kōwa K.K., Nagoya, Japan), or iCare rebound tonometry (Revenio Group Oyj, Vantaa, Finland). When several IOP measurements were obtained per eye, the median value was recorded.

2.1. Surgery

Both metal probe trabeculotomy and 360-degree catheter trabeculotomy were performed by three experienced ophthalmic surgeons (F.G., N.P., and E.M.H.). For both procedures, the conjunctiva was opened either at the limbus (limbus-based conjunctival flap in 67 eyes) or 8-mm posterior of the limbus (fornix-based conjunctival flap in 25 eyes), depending on the state of the conjunctiva. A 3.5-mm × 3.5-mm partial thickness scleral flap was dissected. A second, deeper, and smaller flap of 1.5 mm in width and 3 mm in length was formed to unroof the Schlemm's canal anterior to the scleral spur (as described before by Chin et al. [18]). Before the probe or catheter insertion, acetylcholine (Miochol-E; Bausch & Lomb Inc., Bridgewater, NJ, USA) and a cohesive ophthalmic viscoelastic device (Healon® or Healon®GV; Abbott Laboratories Inc., Abbott Park, IL, USA) were injected into the anterior chamber via a paracentesis to achieve miosis and a deep, stable anterior chamber.

For probe trabeculotomy, the probe was then inserted into one ostium of the Schlemm's canal and gently rotated into the anterior chamber, and this procedure was repeated through the other ostium of Schlemm's canal. In cases where the opening of Schlemm's canal was identified with certainty, no gonioscopic control was performed. However, in some patients, especially in secondary glaucoma patients and in anterior chamber and/or angle anomalies, gonioscopic verification was carried out. For 360-degree trabeculotomy, the illuminated iTRACK microcatheter (iTRACK 250A; iScience Interventional, Menlo Park, CA, USA) was inserted and advanced through the entire circumference of the Schlemm's canal. Once the tip of the catheter appeared in the opposite ostium, both ends were pulled in a purse string manner, thus performing a 360° trabeculotomy. Thereafter, for both procedures, the small, deep, and superficial scleral flaps were closed with single 10-0 nylon lamellar sutures. The conjunctiva was closed either by a 10-0 nylon continuous limbal mattress suture in the cases of fornix-based conjunctival flaps or by a 9-0 vicryl double-layer suture in cases of limbal-based conjunctival flaps.

In cases of combined trabeculectomy with trabeculotomy, the Descemet bridge anterior to the Schlemm's canal was perforated, and a small trabecular block was removed. Small iridectomy was only performed in the case of iris incarceration.

2.2. Outcome Measures

The main outcome measure was long-term IOP development. IOP was recorded by applanation tonometry and by iCare rebound tonometry, if possible, at each visit in both eyes. IOP was analyzed in the following manner: IOP at presentation, at last follow-up or before second operation, and the difference of IOP between presentation and last follow-up or before second operation, as well as the difference in IOP pre- and postoperatively.

Surgical success was defined as IOP < 21 mmHg in eyes without a need for further intervention for pressure reduction. A qualified success was defined as IOP < 21 mmHg requiring pressure-lowering medication.

The axial length (AL) and corneal diameter (CD) were measured under anesthesia using a-scan ultrasonography. The axial length and corneal diameter were recorded at the first examination and at the last examination. Furthermore, the difference of AL between affected and unaffected eyes was compared over the observation period.

2.3. Statistical Analysis

For categorical data, the absolute and relative frequencies were computed. For continuous data, the median and interquartile range were calculated. The primary (IOP) and secondary outcomes (AL and CD) were compared using the Mann–Whitney U test for continuous variables and Wilcoxon signed-rank test for paired analysis. The significance for all analyses was set at $p < 0.05$. The analyses were performed with SPSS version 24 (IBM, Armonk, NY, USA).

3. Results

3.1. Description of the Population

A total of 61 patients were included: 32 patients had bilateral and 29 unilateral congenital glaucoma, resulting in 93 eyes with childhood glaucoma. Thirty-six children with primary congenital glaucoma (PCG), seven children with Sturge-Weber syndrome, seven children with aphakic glaucoma, six with Axenfeld-Rieger syndrome, three patients with Peter's anomaly, and two patients with other anomalies were evaluated. The median follow-up time was 78.2 months (interquartile range: 28.8–122.1 months). The mean age at diagnosis was 3.7 ± 5.1 years. Baseline characteristics are described in Table 1.

Table 1. Baseline characteristics.

Characteristic	Total (n = 61)
Demographic	
Age, Median (IQR), y	1.0 ± (0.1–7.0)
Female sex % (no.)	42.6 (26)
Bilateral glaucoma % (no.)	52.5 (32)
Preop. IOP Median (IQR), mmHg	31.0 (25.25–38.75)
Medication classes, median (IQR)	3.0 (1.0–4.0)
Classification of childhood glaucoma % (no.)	
Primary congenital glaucoma	59.0 (36)
Glaucoma associated with nonacquired systemic disease or syndrome	
Sturge-Weber syndrome	11.5 (7)
Glaucoma associated with nonacquired ocular anomalies	
Aphakia	11.5 (7)
Axenfeld-Rieger syndrome	9.8 (6)
Peter's anomaly	4.9 (3)
Glaucoma associated with nonacquired ocular anomalies	3.2 (2)
Haab striae % (no.)	43.0 (40)

IOP = intraocular pressure; IQR = interquartile range; n = number.

Two hundred and seventy-one glaucoma surgeries were performed on all the included eyes (mean 3.3 ± 3.7 interventions per eye), largely due to the high number of cyclodestructive interventions (see Table 2). The approach of surgical management differed for patients with PCG compared to those with other forms of childhood glaucoma. While the proportion of cyclodestructive interventions was 43% in patients with PCG, it was 69% in the others. Accordingly, incisional surgery accounted for 57% for PCG and only 31% for the other forms of childhood glaucoma.

Table 2. Number of operations.

Total Number of Operations	All	PCG
Controlled cyclophotocoagulation	130	61
Cyclocryotherapy	16	5
Trabeculotomy	52	38
Combined trabeculectomy/trabeculotomy	11	7
Revision after trabeculotomy	9	7
Re-trabeculotomy	24	18
Trabeculectomy	2	0
Aqueous Shunt Implantation	19	12
Revision after filtering surgery	8	7

PCG = primary congenital glaucoma.

3.2. Management and Control of IOP

IOP was obtained at the first and last visits in 84 out of 93 (90%) glaucomatous eyes. Nine eyes with missing data (10%) due to noncompliance of the children at the last visit were excluded from evaluation. Overall, the mean IOP at the first visit was 32.8 ± 10.2 mmHg and decreased to 15.5 ± 7.3 mmHg at the last visit ($p < 0.001$) in all the patients. In the group of PCG patients, IOP from the first visit of 31.2 ± 9.5 decreased to 14.3 ± 5.8 at the last visit ($p < 0.001$).

In the metal probe trabeculotomy (TO) group (52 eyes), IOP decreased from 27.8 ± 8 mmHg to 11.2 ± 4.4 after surgery ($p < 0.001$). In the combined trabeculectomy with trabeculotomy group (11 eyes), the preoperative IOP decreased from 35.8 ± 10.2 mmHg to 11.1 ± 6.2 after operation ($p = 0.003$), as shown in Figure 2a. There was no significant difference for IOP after surgery between the two groups ($p = 0.94$). In the subgroup of PCG, 38 eyes were treated with a TO, reducing the IOP from 28.0 ± 8.4 mmHg to 10.5 ± 3.8 mmHg ($p < 0.001$). Furthermore, in the PCG subgroup, seven eyes were treated with combined trabeculectomy with trabeculotomy, reducing the IOP from 37.3 ± 11.9 mmHg to 8.9 ± 5.4 mmHg ($p < 0.001$), as shown in Figure 2b. The PCG subgroup did not show a significant difference in postoperative IOP between the two procedures ($p = 0.34$).

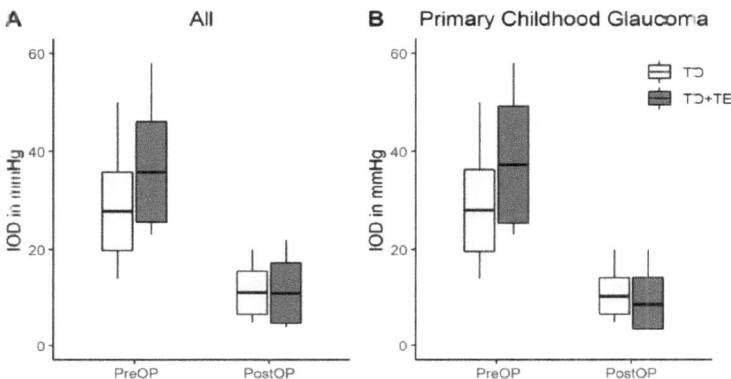

Figure 2. IOP development. IOP values (in mmHg): (**A**) preoperative and postoperative IOP values in all patients (light grey: the metal probe trabeculotomy (TO) group and dark grey: the combined trabeculectomy with trabeculotomy group (TO + TE)) and (**B**) preoperative and postoperative IOP values in the PCG subgroup (light grey: the metal probe trabeculotomy (TO) group and dark grey: the combined trabeculectomy with trabeculotomy group (TO + TE)).

3.3. Postoperative Complications

The most common complication after TO was transient hypotony (IOP < 5 mmHg) in six eyes (12%) and IOP spike (2%), suprachoroidal hemorrhage (2%), and pupillary distortion (2%), each occurring in one eye. After combined trabeculectomy with trabeculotomy, transient hypotony was seen in six eyes (55%); four of these (35%) presented choroidal effusion. There was one case of IOP elevation after combined trabeculectomy with trabeculotomy.

3.4. Success

At the time of the last follow-up, 62% of all eyes that underwent surgery achieved complete surgical success without IOP-lowering medication. Qualified surgical success (with or without additional medication) was reached by 85% of the eyes. In the subgroup of PCG patients, the rate of qualified surgical success was 89%.

3.5 Development of Axial Length (AL) and Corneal Diameter (CD)

The mean AL at the first examination was 22.1 ± 2.2 mm and 23.6 ± 2.9 mm at the last examination. For evaluation of the axial length development, we compared the AL of glaucomatous eyes with the AL of healthy eyes in children with unilateral glaucoma. We did not find a significant difference in axial length growth between glaucoma eyes and normal eyes ($p = 0.3$). When compared, the PCG group showed a significantly higher axial length of 22.6 ± 2.1 mm at the first examination compared to the other forms of childhood glaucoma (21.1 ± 1.8 mm) ($p = 0.02$). At the last examination, this difference was minimized, with an axial length of 23.6 ± 2.5 mm in the PCG group and 23.5 ± 3.6 mm in the other types of childhood glaucoma, respectively ($p = 0.90$).

The mean horizontal CD at the first examination was 12.7 ± 1.3 mm and 13.2 ± 1.1 mm at the last examination. The CD development was compared between glaucomatous and healthy eyes. Over the observed duration, there was no significant difference in CD growth between glaucomatous eyes and healthy eyes ($p = 0.80$). The mean horizontal CD was significantly larger at the first and last examinations in patients with PCG (13.3 ± 1.0 and 13.6 ± 0.9) compared to patients with other forms of childhood glaucoma (11.6 ± 0.8 and 12.4 ± 1.1) ($p < 0.001$).

3.6. Refractive Change

We defined emmetropia as the spherical equivalent within $+/-1$ dpt, with values below that as myopia and above as hyperopia. Using this definition, 15% of all glaucomatous eyes were emmetropic, 60% myopic, and 25% hyperopic at the baseline. At the end of the study, 16% were emmetropic, 58% myopic, and 26% hyperopic. In healthy contralateral eyes of unilateral glaucoma, 31% showed emmetropia, 8% myopia, and 61% hyperopia at the baseline vs. 54% emmetropia, 23% myopia, and 23% hyperopia at the last examination, respectively. The refractive status of the eyes with PCG and glaucoma of other types is shown separately in Table 3. The rate of myopia was significantly higher in the group of PCG both at the beginning and at the end ($p < 0.01$).

Table 3. Refractive status in eyes with primary childhood glaucoma (PCG) (upper line) and eyes with other forms of childhood glaucoma than PCG (lower line) at the baseline and end of follow-up.

PCG	Baseline			End of Follow-Up		
	Emmetropia	Hyperopia	Myopia	Emmetropia	Hyperopia	Myopia
Yes	8%	18%	74%	18%	13%	68%
No	29%	41%	29%	12%	53%	35%

4. Discussion

In this study, we evaluated the long-term data of childhood glaucoma in terms of various parameters, such as corneal diameter, refraction, axial length, and intraocular pressure, in 61 children. Furthermore, we analyzed the number and the various types of surgeries performed in children with glaucoma at the University Medical Center, Mainz, Germany. Our study population was heterogeneous with respect to the different forms of childhood glaucoma. The most common entity of childhood glaucoma among our patients was primary congenital glaucoma (PCG), which mirrors its higher prevalence [3,4]; therefore, we paid special attention to the results of this subgroup.

The preoperative IOP in our study cohort was 32.8 ± 10.2 mmHg and was therefore similar to those described by other studies for comparable cohorts of children with glaucoma (29.1–31.5 mmHg) [19–21]. We found an IOP reduction of 14.3 ± 5.8 mmHg, which is comparable to the existing literature (values between 11.07 and 17.0 mmHg) [5,21,22].

For surgical success, we chose 21 mmHg as our cut-off value, according to the guidelines. However, it should be discussed whether this cut-off-value is sufficient enough for a heterogeneous patient cohort. Most studies have used similar IOP values [5,23], while some authors used higher cut-off values of up to 24 mmHg [24]. The debate about success after glaucoma surgery and its often arbitrarily chosen IOP end points is currently underway, with differing viewpoints concerning the ideal IOP cut-off value [25]. Comparisons of success after glaucoma surgery should therefore take the varying criteria of success into account. We observed a complete surgical success rate, without IOP-lowering medication, of 62% and a rate of 85% for qualified success, where patients with or without IOP-lowering medication were counted as successes. These values are comparable to studies with similar cohorts of patients that also chose a cut-off of 21 mmHg for surgical success, where success rates of 79.5–80.4% were reported [5,26]. However, our somewhat lower success rates can, in part, be explained by the high proportion of secondary childhood glaucoma cases in our population. Patients with secondary childhood glaucoma often have a more advanced disease and do require repeated surgeries, as seen in our cohort. Comparing combined trabeculotomy–trabeculectomy [27,28] vs. trabeculotomy alone, higher preoperative IOP values were present in patients who received the combination operation (35.8 ± 10.2 mmHg) compared to those with standalone trabeculotomy (27.8 ± 8 mmHg). The IOP decreased to almost equal values of 11.2 in the TE + TO group and 11.1 in the TO group, respectively. When only the PCG collective was considered, analogous results were obtained. Khalil et al. compared these two methods in patients with primary congenital glaucoma and reported similar results of 11.1 mmHg for TO and 11.3 mmHg for combined trabeculectomy with trabeculotomy one month after surgery with a baseline IOP of 24 mmHg [29].

The most common surgical side effect was hemorrhage in eyes that underwent trabeculotomy or TO/TE (19.7% and 37.5%, respectively). Since hemorrhage is an expected event in any kind of trabeculotomy, it is not considered a complication. The reported incidences correspond to the values published by other authors (23–34%) [22,29–31].

The high count of surgical interventions of 3.3 ± 3.7 per eye is largely due to the high number of cyclodestructive interventions (130 out of 271), which was considerably higher in patients with other forms of childhood glaucoma than PCG (69%) compared to those with PCG (43%). Our cohort received a high number of controlled cyclophotocoagulations. In this modified version of cyclophotocoagulation, laser radiation reflected from the fundus is recorded by a photodetector outside the eye. The time dependence of this detector signal directly monitors the change in transmission of the coagulated tissue; with this information, the surgeon or a computer can interrupt the laser process [32]. The surgical approaches at our clinic have changed over the last ten years. Formerly, cyclodestructive techniques were applied frequently, particularly in secondary glaucoma but, also, in primary congenital glaucoma. This approach has been changed in the last few years, as 360° trabeculotomy and probe trabeculotomy have become the standard of care in childhood glaucoma in our clinic [33,34]. One has to bear in mind that the observation time of this study started in 1995, when other surgical techniques and experience were applied in our clinic. In a similar study, Alsheikheh et al. reported 2.5 interventions per eye during an observation period over 5 years [22]. Zetterberg et al. reported a mean of 2.3 pressure-lowering interventions in an average period of 5.9 years, including a number of cyclophotocoagulations [20].

Various authors consider the axial length an important criterion for the diagnosis and follow-up of childhood glaucoma [35–37]. A significant growth of the axial length was found at the first (22.4 ± 2.2 mm) and the last measurements (23.9 + 2.9 mm) of all the eyes, corresponding to physiological elongation. In children with unilateral glaucomatous eyes and healthy eyes, no significant difference in AL growth was seen over the observed period ($p = 0.3$). Kiefer et al. and Mayer et al. reported similar AL values of 22.5 mm preoperatively, 24.2 mm postoperatively and 22.3 mm preoperatively, 23.9 mm postoperatively, respectively [23,26].

Kiskis et al. [38] considered the corneal diameter to be more reliable than the axial length in childhood glaucoma. In our study, however, we could not find a significant difference in corneal diameters between the first and the last visits. Although changes of the corneal diameter may provide some additional information during follow-up of childhood glaucoma, small changes of the corneal diameter are difficult to detect. Thus, axial length changes remain an important morphological parameter in monitoring the progress of glaucoma. Indeed, surgical decisions are not made solely on the basis of IOP but, also, on the basis of AL.

Another important clinical factor is the refractive error [39–41]. The baseline prevalence of myopia in our study (60%) corresponds well to other reports [26,42–44]. Hyperopia is reported heterogenous in the literature, and the prevalence in our study (25%) corresponds well to the publications by Dannheim [44], Mandel [42], and Meyer [26], who reported prevalences of 22.9, 25.6, and 33.3%, respectively, while Schlieter [43] and Alsheikheh [22] reported lower rates of 11.5% and 0% of hyperopia of more than 1 diopter, respectively. As the refractive error is known to be a valuable indicator of operative success or disease progression [39], the fact that there was no further myopization of the cohort after surgical intervention may be considered positive.

We saw significantly higher myopia rates, corneal diameters, and axial lengths at the first examination in eyes with PCG compared to other forms of childhood glaucoma, which is not surprising considering that buphthalmos is one of the defining diagnostic criteria for PCG. Therefore, myopia, enlarged corneal diameters and axial lengths above the age-appropriate average may be used as indications of PCG in patients with childhood glaucoma.

This study had several limitations. The retrospective study design limited the evaluation of all the clinical parameters; many parameters were only collected when it was therapeutically and diagnostically useful. Moreover, childhood glaucoma, already rare as such, encompasses a wide spectrum of even rarer disorders. Therefore, due to the small number of cases, it was not possible to analyze most subgroups separately, with the exception of PCG. Comparisons between PCG and glaucoma of other types are of limited validity, as the latter group consists of a diverse spectrum of anomalies. However, reasonable data on childhood glaucoma are rare in the literature, and we believe that our data can add some insight into the treatment of glaucoma in newborns and children.

This study summarizes the treatment of childhood glaucoma over the last two decades until 2015. In conclusion, our results showed the positive results of surgical intervention and underlie the necessity of early and sufficient treatment for childhood glaucoma in specialized centers. However, the treatment has changed since 2015; nowadays, circumferential catheter-assisted trabeculotomy is the main method of choice in our center.

Since research on childhood glaucoma mainly consists of retrospective studies with smaller cohorts, there is a need for a standardized examination protocol and documentation of pediatric glaucoma, such as a childhood glaucoma database, that could improve the care for children with glaucoma.

Author Contributions: Conceptualization, E.M.H.; methodology, E.M.H. and F.M.W.; software, A.K.-G.S. and F.M.W.; validation, E.M.H., J.V.S., A.K.-G.S., N.P., and F.G.; formal analysis, L.U., F.M.W., J.V.S., and A.K.-G.S.; investigation, L.U. and E.M.H.; resources, N.P. and E.M.H.; data curation, L.U. and F.M.W.; writing—original draft preparation, F.M.W. and E.M.H.; writing—review and editing, E.M.H., J.V.S., A.K.-G.S., N.P., and F.G.; visualization, L.U. and F.M.W.; supervision, E.M.H.; project administration, E.M.H.; and funding acquisition, E.M.H. All authors have read and agreed to the published version of the manuscript.

Funding: This research received no external funding.

Institutional Review Board Statement: This study was conducted according to the guidelines of the Declaration of Helsinki. Ethical review and approval were waived for this study, according to the regional laws.

Informed Consent Statement: According to the regional laws, the requirement for informed consent was waived by the ethics committee of the medical board.

Data Availability Statement: The data presented in this study are available on request from the corresponding author. The data are not publicly available due to their containing information that could compromise the privacy of research participants.

Conflicts of Interest: The authors declare no conflict of interest.

References

1. Thau, A.; Lloyd, M.; Freedman, S.; Beck, A.; Grajewski, A.; Levin, A.V. New classification system for pediatric glaucoma: Implications for clinical care and a research registry. *Curr. Opin. Ophthalmol.* **2018**, *29*, 385–394. [CrossRef] [PubMed]
2. Beck, A.; Chang, T.; Freedman, S. Definition, Classification, Differential Diagnosis. In Proceedings of the 9th Consensus Meeting: Childhood Glaucoma, Vancouver, BC, Canada, 16 July 2013; Weinreb, R.N., Grajewski, A., Papadopoulos, M., Grigg, J., Freedman, S., Eds.; Kugler: Amsterdam, The Netherlands, 2013.
3. Papadopoulos, M.; Cable, N.; Rahi, J.; Khaw, P.T.; BIG Eye Study Investigators. The British Infantile and Childhood Glaucoma (BIG) Eye Study. *Investig. Ophthalmol. Vis. Sci.* **2007**, *48*, 4100–4106. [CrossRef] [PubMed]
4. Khan, A.O. Genetics of primary glaucoma. *Curr. Opin. Ophthalmol.* **2011**, *22*, 347–355. [CrossRef] [PubMed]
5. Yassin, S.A.; Al-Tamimi, E.R. Surgical outcomes in children with primary congenital glaucoma: A 20-year experience. *Eur. J. Ophthalmol.* **2016**, *26*, 581–587. [CrossRef] [PubMed]

6. Lotufo, D.; Ritch, R.; Szmyd, L., Jr.; Burris, J.E. Juvenile Glaucoma, Race, and Refraction. *JAMA* **1989**, *261*, 249–252. [CrossRef] [PubMed]
7. Robin, A.L.; Quigley, H.A.; Pollack, I.P.; Edward Maumenee, A.; Maumenee, I.H. An Analysis of Visual Acuity Visual Fields, and Disk Cupping in Childhood Glaucoma. *Am. J. Ophthalmol.* **1979**, *88*, 847–858. [CrossRef]
8. Taylor, R.H.; Ainsworth, J.R.; Evans, A.R.; Levin, A.V. The epidemiology of pediatric glaucoma: The Toronto experience. *J. AAPOS* **1999**, *3*, 308–315. [CrossRef]
9. Chen, T.C.; Chen, P.P.; Francis, B.A.; Junk, A.K.; Smith, S.D.; Singh, K.; Lin, S.C. Pediatric glaucoma surgery: A report by the American Academy of Ophthalmology. *Ophthalmology* **2014**, *121*, 2107–2115. [CrossRef] [PubMed]
10. Morales, J.; Al Shahwan, S.; Al Odhayb, S.; Al Jadaan, I.; Edward, D.P. Current surgical options for the management of pediatric glaucoma. *J. Ophthalmol.* **2013**, *2013*, 763735. [CrossRef] [PubMed]
11. Burian, H.M. A case of Marfan's syndrome with bilateral glaucoma. With description of a new type of operation for developmental glaucoma (trabeculotomy ab externo). *Am. J. Ophthalmol.* **1960**, *50*, 1187–1192. [CrossRef]
12. Smith, R. A new technique for opening the canal of Schlemm. Preliminary report. *Br. J. Ophthalmol.* **1960**, *44*, 370–373. [CrossRef] [PubMed]
13. Chang, T.C.; Cavuoto, K.M. Surgical management in primary congenital glaucoma: Four debates. *J. Ophthalmol.* **2013**, *2013*, 612708. [CrossRef]
14. Dietlein, T.S. Glaucoma surgery in children. *Ophthalmologe* **2015**, *112*, 95–101. [CrossRef]
15. Harms, H.; Dannheim, R. Erfahrungen mit der trabekulotomia ab externo beim angebore-nen Glaukom. *3er. Dtsch Ophthalmol. Ges.* **1969**, *69*, 272.
16. Papadopoulos, M.; Edmunds, B.; Fenerty, C.; Khaw, P.T. Childhood glaucoma surgery in the 21st century. *Eye* **2014**, *28*, 931–943. [CrossRef] [PubMed]
17. Chang, I.; Capricli, J.; Ou, Y. Surgical Management of Pediatric Glaucoma. *Dev. Ophthalmol.* **2017**, *59*, 165–178. [CrossRef] [PubMed]
18. Chin, S.; Nitta, T.; Shinmei, Y.; Aoyagi, M.; Nitta, A.; Ohno, S.; Ishida, S.; Yoshida, K. Reduction of intraocular pressure using a modified 360-degree suture trabeculotomy technique in primary and secondary open-angle glaucoma: A pilot study. *J. Glaucoma* **2012**, *21*, 401–407. [CrossRef] [PubMed]
19. Bussieres, J.F.; Therrien, R.; Hamel, P.; Barret, P.; Prot-Labarthe, S. Retrospective cohort study of 163 pediatric glaucoma patients. *Can. J. Ophthalmol.* **2009**, *44*, 323–327. [CrossRef] [PubMed]
20. Zetterberg, M.; Nystrom, A.; Kalaboukhova, L.; Magnusson, G. Outcome of surgical treatment of primary and secondary glaucoma in young children. *Acta Ophthalmol.* **2015**, *93*, 269–275. [CrossRef] [PubMed]
21. Aponte, E.P.; Diehl, N.; Mohney, B.G. Medical and surgical outcomes in childhood glaucoma: A population-based study. *J. AAPOS* **2011**, *15*, 263–267. [CrossRef] [PubMed]
22. Alsheikheh, A.; Klink, J.; Klirk, T.; Steffen, H.; Grehn, F. Long-term results of surgery in childhood glaucoma. *Graefes Arch. Clin. Exp. Ophthalmol.* **2007**, *245*, 195–203. [CrossRef] [PubMed]
23. Kiefer, G.; Schwenn, O.; Grehn, F. Correlation of postoperative axial length growth and intraocular pressure in congenital glaucoma—A retrospective study in trabeculotomy and goniotomy. *Graefes Arch. Clin. Exp. Ophthalmol.* **2001**, *239*, 893–899. [CrossRef] [PubMed]
24. Areaux, R.G.; Grajewski, A.L.; Balasubramaniam, S.; Brandt, J.D.; Jun, A.; Edmunds, B.; Shyne, M.T.; Bitrian, E. Trabeculotomy Ab Interno with the Trab360 Device for Childhood Glaucomas. *Am. J. Ophthalmol.* **2020**, *209*, 178–186. [CrossRef] [PubMed]
25. Rotchford, A.P.; King, A.J. Moving the goal posts definitions of success after glaucoma surgery and their effect on reported outcome. *Ophthalmology* **2010**, *117*, 18–23.e3. [CrossRef]
26. Meyer, G.; Schwenn, O.; Pfeiffer, N.; Grehn, F. Trabeculotomy in congenital glaucoma. *Graefes Arch. Clin. Exp. Ophthalmol.* **2000**, *238*, 207–213. [CrossRef] [PubMed]
27. Mandal, A.K.; Matalia, J.H.; Nutheti, R.; Krishnaiah, S. Combined trabeculotomy and trabeculectomy in advanced primary developmental glaucoma with corneal diameter of 14 mm or more. *Eye* **2006**, *20*, 135–143. [CrossRef]
28. Mandal, A.K.; Naduvilath, T.J.; Jayagandan, A. Surgical results of combined trabeculotomy-trabeculectomy for developmental glaucoma. *Ophthalmology* **1998**, *105*, 974–982. [CrossRef]
29. Khalil, D.H.; Abdelhakim, M.A. Primary trabeculotomy compared to combined trabeculectomy-trabeculotomy in congenital glaucoma: 3-year study. *Acta Ophthalmol.* **2016**, *94*, e550–e554. [CrossRef]
30. McPherson, S.D., Jr.; Berry, D.P. Goniotomy vs external trabeculotomy for developmental glaucoma. *Am. J. Ophthalmol.* **1983**, *95*, 427–431. [CrossRef]
31. McPherson, S.D., Jr.; McFarland, D. External trabeculotomy for developmental glaucoma. *Ophthalmology* **1980**, *87*, 302–305. [CrossRef]
32. Preußner, P.-R.; Boos, N.; Faßbender, K.; Schwenn, O.; Pfeiffer, N. Real-time control for transscleral cyclophotocoagulation. *Graefe's Arch. Clin. Exp. Ophthalmol.* **1997**, *235*, 794–801. [CrossRef] [PubMed]
33. Hoffmann, E.M.; Aghayeva, F.; Schuster, A.K.; Pfeiffer, N.; Karsten, M.; Schweiger, S.; Pirlich, N.; Wagner, F.M.; Chronopoulos, P.; Grehn, F. Results of childhood glaucoma surgery over a long-term period. *Acta Ophthalmol.* **2021**. [CrossRef]
34. Hoffmann, E.M. 360° trabeculotomy for pediatric glaucoma. *Ophthalmologe* **2020**, *117*, 210–214. [CrossRef] [PubMed]

35. Buschmann, W.; Bluth, K. Regular echographic axial measurements of the eye in controlling intraocular pressure regulation in hydrophthalmos. *Klin. Mon. Augenheilkd.* **1974**, *165*, 878–886.
36. Dietlein, T.S.; Jacobi, P.C.; Krieglstein, G.K. Eyeball growth after successful glaucoma surgery in the 1st year of life–follow-up values for primary congenital glaucoma. *Klin. Mon. Augenheilkd.* **1998**, *213*, 67–70. [CrossRef] [PubMed]
37. Sampaolesi, R.; Caruso, R. Ocular echometry in the diagnosis of congenital glaucoma. *Arch. Ophthalmol.* **1982**, *100*, 574–577. [CrossRef] [PubMed]
38. Kiskis, A.A.; Markowitz, S.N.; Morin, J.D. Corneal diameter and axial length in congenital glaucoma. *Can. J. Ophthalmol.* **1985**, *20*, 93–97. [PubMed]
39. Broughton, W.L.; Parks, M.M. An Analysis of Treatment of Congenital Glaucoma by Goniotomy. *Am. J. Ophthalmol.* **1981**, *91*, 566–572. [CrossRef]
40. Douglas, D.H. Reflections on buphthalmos and goniotomy. *Trans. Ophthalmol. Soc.* **1970**, *90*, 931–937.
41. Haas, J. Principles and Problems of Therapy in Congenital Glaucoma. *Investig. Ophthalmol. Vis. Sci.* **1968**, *7*, 140–146.
42. Mandal, A.K.; Gothwal, V.K.; Bagga, H.; Nutheti, R.; Mansoori, T. Outcome of surgery on infants younger than 1 month with congenital glaucoma. *Ophthalmology* **2003**, *110*, 1909–1915. [CrossRef]
43. Schlieter, F.; Nathrath, P.; Nicolai, R. Follow-up examination long after surgical treatment of congenital glaucomas (author's transl). *Klin. Mon. Augenheilkd.* **1974**, *164*, 317–320.
44. Dannheim, R.; Haas, H. Visual acuity and intraocular pressure after surgery in congenital glaucoma (author's transl). *Klin. Mon. Augenheilkd.* **1980**, *177*, 296–303. [CrossRef] [PubMed]

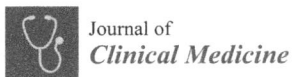

Article

The Efficacy, Safety and Satisfaction Associated with Switching from Brinzolamide 1% and Brimonidine 0.1% to a Fixed Combination of Brinzolamide 1% and Brimonidine 0.1% in Glaucoma Patients

Hiromitsu Onoe [1], Kazuyuki Hirooka [1,*], Mikio Nagayama [2], Atsushi Hirota [3], Hideki Mochizuki [4], Takeshi Sagara [5], Katsuyoshi Suzuki [6], Hideaki Okumichi [1] and Yoshiaki Kiuchi [1]

[1] Department of Ophthalmology and Visual Science, Hiroshima University, Hiroshima 734-8551, Japan; onoehir@hiroshima-u.ac.jp (H.O.); onmic@hiroshima-u.ac.jp (H.O.); ykiuchi@hiroshima-u.ac.jp (Y.K.)
[2] Nagayama Eye Clinic, Okayama 714-0086, Japan; mikio@po.harenet.ne.jp
[3] Hirota Eye Clinic, Yamaguchi 745-0017, Japan; hirotaganka@lion.ocn.ne.jp
[4] Kusatsu Eye Clinic, Hiroshima 733-0861, Japan; mochizuki-h@hiroshima-u.ac.jp
[5] Sagara Eye Clinic, Yamaguchi 758-0021, Japan; tsagara@sagara-eye.jp
[6] Suzuki Eye Clinic, Yamaguchi 755-0155, Japan; suzuki_eye@grace.ocn.ne.jp
* Correspondence: khirooka9@gmail.com; Tel.: +81-82-257-5247; Fax: +81-82-257-5249

Abstract: We evaluated glaucoma patients for the efficacy, safety and satisfaction associated with switching from brinzolamide 1% and brimonidine 0.1% to a fixed combination of brinzolamide 1% and brimonidine 0.1%. A total of 22 glaucoma patients were enrolled and completed this prospective, nonrandomized study that evaluated patients who underwent treatment with at least brinzolamide 1% and brimonidine 0.1%. Patients on brinzolamide 1% and brimonidine 0.1% were switched to a brinzolamide/brimonidine fixed-combination ophthalmic suspension (BBFC). Evaluations of intraocular pressure (IOP), superficial punctate keratopathy (SPK) and conjunctival hyperemia were conducted at baseline and at 4 and 12 weeks. The Treatment Satisfaction Questionnaire for Medication-9 (TSQM-9) was utilized to assess the change in treatment satisfaction. At baseline and at 4 and 12 weeks, the IOP was 15.0 ± 4.1, 14.8 ± 4.1 and 14.8 ± 4.1 mmHg, respectively. There were no significant differences observed at any of the time points. However, the SPK score significantly decreased at 12 weeks, even though no significant differences were observed for the conjunctival hyperemia incidence at any of the time points. After switching from brinzolamide 1% and brimonidine 0.1% to BBFC, there was a significant increase in the TSQM-9 score for convenience and global satisfaction. Both an improvement in the degree of SPK and an increase in treatment satisfaction occurred after switching from brinzolamide 1% and brimonidine 0.1% to BBFC, even though there were sustained IOP values throughout the 12-week evaluation period.

Keywords: glaucoma; brinzolamide; brimonidine; satisfaction

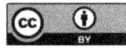

1. Introduction

The degeneration of retinal ganglion cells that results in visual field loss can potentially lead to blindness, and is the primary characteristic of the progressive optic neuropathy that is referred to as glaucoma [1]. The key risk factor for the development and progression of glaucomatous neuropathy is an elevated intraocular pressure (IOP) [2]. Methods for reducing the glaucoma progression risk have been reported by several studies and have all been associated with a lowering of the IOP [3,4].

In order to achieve successful glaucoma management, the use of combination therapy with multiple IOP-lowering medications is suggested when monotherapy proves to be insufficient [5]. Although lowering of the IOP can be achieved through the use of multiple medications, decreased patient adherence to treatment and persistence with the therapy can limit the effectiveness of the treatment [6,7]. However, when fixed combinations are utilized so that a single formulation contains two or more medications, this helps to reduce the dosing frequency in addition to reducing the exposure of patients to preservatives. Therefore, this suggests that improvements in both patient comfort and the adherence to and persistence of the treatment could potentially be achieved when using fixed-dose combinations [8,9].

At the present time, the only fixed-combination glaucoma therapy that does not contain a β-blocker is the brinzolamide/brimonidine fixed-combination ophthalmic suspension. Several studies have reported that the administration of BBFC two to three times daily in open-angle glaucoma (OAG) or patients with ocular hypertension that were adequately controlled with prostaglandin analogs led to an effective lowering of the IOP [10–12]. In Japan, the administration of BBFC two times daily was approved for use in 2019.

The current study aimed to evaluate the switching of patients from brinzolamide 1% and brimonidine 0.1% to BBFC, and then investigate the efficacy, safety and satisfaction associated with this change. After the switch in these medications, this meant that patients only needed to use one bottle of eye drops with an instillation of two drops per day, which was much simpler as compared to their previous procedures.

2. Materials and Methods

From October 2020 to August 2021, six investigational sites participated in this clinical trial. These sites included Hiroshima University Hospital (Hiroshima, Japan), Nagayama Eye Clinic (Okayama, Japan), Hirota Eye Clinic (Yamaguchi, Japan), Sagara Eye Clinic (Yamaguchi, Japan), Kusatsu Eye Clinic (Hiroshima, Japan) and Suzuki Eye Clinic (Yamaguchi, Japan). The Institutional Review Board of Hiroshima University approved the study protocol. All subjects provided written informed consent for participation in the research study in accordance with the principles outlined in the Declaration of Helsinki.

All patients underwent examinations of visual acuity, refraction, visual field, slit-lamp examination and gonioscopy. Eligibility criteria included an age ≥ 20 years, glaucomatous optic disc abnormalities and corresponding glaucomatous visual field defects, in addition to being treated with at least brinzolamide 1% (Alcon Laboratories Inc, Ft Worth, TX, USA; preservative: 0.005% sodium chloride) and brimonidine 0.1% (Senju Pharmaceutical Co. Ltd., Osaka, Japan; preservative: 0.01% benzalkonium chloride). Exclusion criteria included subjects having active ocular diseases in either eye with the exception of glaucoma, having retinal disease with a potential risk of progression, having undergone ocular surgery or laser treatment within the previous 1 year, being on a regimen for systemic or local administration of steroids during this study or having corneal disease in either eye that potentially posed a problem for accurate IOP measurements. If both eyes of a patient met the inclusion criteria, the analysis used the eye with the higher IOP. When the IOP was the same in both eyes, the analysis used the right eye.

Patient examinations during the study consisted of 3 scheduled visits that occurred over 12 weeks (day 0 and weeks 4 and 12). At day 0 (baseline), patients deemed eligible for enrollment and who were using brinzolamide 1% and brimonidine 0.1% were switched to BBFC (Senju Pharmaceutical Co. Ltd., Osaka, Japan; preservative: 0.003% benzalkonium chloride).

At each visit, patients underwent measurements for IOP, best-correlated visual acuity and biomicroscopic examinations. Using a Goldmann applanation tonometer, with the same procedure performed at all centers, the IOP was measured during the same time as the brinzolamide 1% and brimonidine 0.1% administration. The primary efficacy outcome was defined as the main change in the IOP at 12 weeks from the baseline. Prior to switching to BBFC, the average baseline IOP was determined twice before implementing any changes.

For biomicroscopy, all patients underwent a slit-lamp examination. To assess the conjunctival hyperemia, we used a 4-point hyperemia grading scale that utilized four different photographs to determine the hyperemia matching. These included: 0 = no hyperemia, 1 = slight hyperemia, 2 = moderate hyperemia and 3 = severe hyperemia. Recording of the corneal epithelial disorders during the slit-lamp examination used an A (area) D (density) grading scale [13].

The Treatment Satisfaction Questionnaire for Medication-9 (TSQM-9) was used to assess the change in treatment statisfaction [14]. The TSQM-9 uses a 5- or 7-point scale to determine the assessment, with an increase in the scores indicating there is an increase in the treatment satisfaction. These results can be further grouped in order to indicate the effectiveness, convenience and global satisfaction scores. For these three evaluated areas, the total scores can range from 0 to 100. Greater satisfaction is equated with a higher total score. All patients completed the questionnaires at baseline and again at 12 weeks.

For continuous variables, the Anderson–Darling test was used to assess the variance equality. Based on the results obtained, differences between the baseline and follow-up visits were then assessed by either a Student's *t*-test or Wilcoxon signed-rank test. Scores for the TSQM-9 are presented as the median and interquartile ranges. All statistical analyses were conducted using JMP software version 15 (SAS Inc., Cary, NC, USA). Statistical significance was indicated by a P value of 0.05 or less. All data are presented as the mean ± standard deviation.

3. Results

This study evaluated a total of 22 patients (22 eyes), with all of the patients completing 12 weeks of follow-up. Baseline patient demographic data are shown in Table 1. The mean age was 67.2 ± 17.2 years.

Table 1. Baseline patient characteristics.

Age (years)	67.2 ± 17.2
Gender (M/F)	12/10
Untreated IOP (mmHg)	20.9 ± 6.0
Baseline IOP (mmHg)	15.0 ± 4.1
Mean deviation (dB)	−10.6 ± 10.0
Type of glaucoma	
POAG	14
NTG	5
Exfoliation glaucoma	3
IOP-lowering medications	
(except brimonidine and brinzolamide)	
PGA	15
PGA/β-blocker	5
None	1

M: male; F: female; IOP: intraocular pressure; POAG: primary open-angle glaucoma; NTG: normal-tension glaucoma; PGA: prostaglandin analogue.

At baseline, the IOP was 15.0 ± 4.1 mmHg, while at 4 weeks it was 14.8 ± 4.1 mmHg and 14.8 ± 4.1 mmHg at 12 weeks (Figure 1). No significant differences were observed between the baseline and each of the follow-up visits. Table 2 presents the degree of SPK that was assessed when using the AD grading scale along with the conjunctival hyperemia scores. Although there was no difference between baseline and the 12-week values for the conjunctival hyperemia score, significant improvement was noted for the degree of SPK at 12 weeks.

Comparison of the baseline TSQM-9 scores indicated that patients were satisfied with both the treatment and its convenience. However, there was no significant difference found with regard to the effectiveness (Table 3).

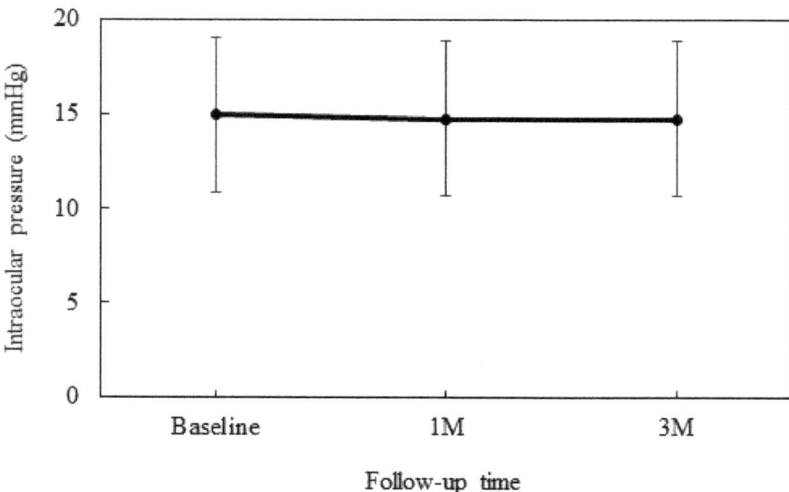

Figure 1. Mean intraocular pressure at baseline and at 4 and 12 weeks. There was no significant difference observed in the mean IOP as compared to the baseline.

Table 2. SPK and hyperemia score.

	SPK Score	p Value *	Hyperemia Score	p Value *
Baseline	1.18 ± 1.26		0.43 ± 0.75	
1M	0.83 ± 1.10	0.40	0.61 ± 0.85	0.33
3M	0.55 ± 0.92	0.02	0.48 ± 0.75	0.58

SPK; superficial punctate keratopathy; * Calculated using Wilcoxon signed-rank test.

Table 3. TSQM-9 scores.

	Baseline (IQR)	3M (IQR)	p Value *
Effectiveness	61 (49–68)	67 (50–72)	0.10
Convenience	67 (50–79)	72 (67–85)	0.01
Global satisfaction	71 (62–79)	79 (69–93)	0.02

IQR: interquartile range. * Calculated using Wilcoxon signed-rank test.

4. Discussion

Throughout the 12-week observation period, the IOP values and conjunctival hyperemia were sustained after switching to BBFC from brinzolamide 1% and brimonidine 0.1%. However, there was a significant improvement in the superficial punctate keratopathy and global satisfaction.

Gandolfi et al. [15] examined patients with OAG or ocular hypertension and reported that BBFC as compared to the concomitant administration of an unfixed combination of brinzolamide 1% and brimonidine 0.2% exhibited an IOP-lowering efficacy. When compared to baseline values, the diurnal IOP change at 3 months was −8.5 ± 0.16 mmHg for patients administered BBFC, while it was −8.3 ± 0.16 mmHg for patients administered brinzolamide and brimonidine. Moreover, a similar IOP-lowering efficacy was found for BBFC as compared to that for brinzolamide and brimonidine. While in Japan a 0.1% concentration of brimonidine is currently used, European countries and North America use 0.2% solutions. Brimonidine concentrations used in Japan were determined based on the results of a dose–response trial that evaluated the IOP-lowering efficacy for Japanese subjects. Therefore, when BBFC is administered in Japan, the formulation uses 0.1%

brimonidine. During the 12-week observation period in our current study, a sustained IOP was observed after switching to BBFC from brinzolamide and brimonidine.

Both the ocular surface and tear balance are known to be affected by IOP-lowering medications [16]. Furthermore, it should be noted that when using 0.1% brimonidine, it contains 0.01% benzalkonium chloride (BAC) as the preservative, while BBFC contains 0.003% BAC as the preservative. A previous study reported that BAC concentrations higher than 0.01% were associated with toxicity on human corneal epithelial cell sheets [17]. In contrast, 1% brinzolamide does not contain BAC, with 0.005% sodium chloride ($NaClO_2$) used as the preservative. A further study that examined corneal epithelial cells following a 30-min exposure to 0.002–0.1% $NaClO_2$ reported finding a high survival rate of 80% or greater [18]. Therefore, these results suggest that $NaClO_2$ causes relatively little corneal damage. Thus, due to the difference in the BAC concentrations between BBFC and 0.1% brimonidine, there was a significant decrease in the AD grading scale observed after switching to BBFC.

When assessing patients' satisfaction with treatments, TSQM-9 has proven to be a reliable instrument, with this questionnaire used for treatment satisfaction assessments in various diseases [14,19,20]. Based on these findings, our current study also used the TSQM-9 to assess patient satisfaction. Another benefit of switching to BBFC from brinzolamide and brimonidine is that there was a reduction in both the number of bottles and instillations. After this switch, the previous two bottles of eye drops and instillation of four drops per day were reduced to one bottle of eye drops and an instillation of only two drops per day. Therefore, the results of our current study demonstrated there was an increase in convenience from the baseline 67 to 72 along with a global satisfaction increase from 71 to 79. Other previous studies have also found that there was a low persistence associated with glaucoma medications when patients were required to use multiple medications [7,21,22]. These results suggest that fixed-combination therapies, including BBFC, can potentially alleviate these types of issues.

There were some limitations for the current study. First, only a relatively small number of cases were evaluated in this study. Therefore, multi-center and larger scale trials will need to be undertaken in order to obtain more rigorous, comparative and definitive evidence and data. One other limitation of our current study was that the observation period used was not long enough. Thus, more clear and definitive results could potentially be obtained when using a longer observation period.

In conclusion, both a sustained IOP along with a significant improvement in the degree of SPK were obtained when switching to BBFC from brinzolamide 1% and brimonidine 0.1%. Furthermore, after switching to BBFC, patients who required multiple IOP-lowering medications reported an improved satisfaction with their medical treatment.

Author Contributions: Conceptualization, K.H.; methodology, K.H.; software, H.O. (Hiromitsu Onoe); validation, H.O. (Hiromitsu Onoe), H.O. (Hideaki Okumichi), M.N., A.H., H.M., T.S., K.S. and Y.K.; formal analysis, H.O. (Hiromitsu Onoe); investigation, H.O. (Hiromitsu Onoe); resources, K.H.; data curation, H.O. (Hiromitsu Onoe); writing—original draft preparation, K.H ; writing—review and editing, K.H.; visualization, K.H.; supervision, K.H.; project administration, K.H.; funding acquisition, K.H. All authors have read and agreed to the published version of the manuscript.

Funding: This research was funded by a Grant-in-Aid for Scientific Research from the Ministry of Education, Culture, Sports, Science, and Technology of Japan (20K09827).

Institutional Review Board Statement: The study was conducted according to the guidelines of the Declaration of Helsinki, and approved by the Institutional Review Board of Hiroshima University (protocol code E-2184 and date of approval).

Informed Consent Statement: Informed consent was obtained from all subjects involved in the study.

Data Availability Statement: The data analyzed in this study are available from the corresponding author on reasonable request.

Conflicts of Interest: The authors declare no conflict of interest.

References

1. Casson, R.J.; Chidlow, G.; Wood, J.P.; Crowston, J.G.; Goldberg, I. Definition of glaucoma: Clinical and experimental concepts. *Clin. Exp. Ophthalmol.* **2012**, *40*, 341–349. [CrossRef]
2. Coleman, A.L.; Miglior, S. Risk factors for glaucoma onset and progression. *Surv. Ophthalmol.* **2008**, *53*, S3–S10. [CrossRef] [PubMed]
3. Leske, M.C.; Heijl, A.; Hussein, M.; Bengtsson, B.; Hyman, L.; Komaroff, E. Early Manifest Glaucoma Trial Group. Factors for glaucoma progression and the effect of treatment: The early manifest glaucoma trial. *Arch. Ophthalmol.* **2003**, *121*, 48–56. [CrossRef] [PubMed]
4. Kass, M.A.; Heuer, D.K.; Higginbotham, E.J.; Johnson, C.A.; Keltner, J.L.; Miller, J.P.; Parrish, R.K.; Wilson, M.R., II; Gordon, M.O. The Ocular Hypertension Treatment Study: A randomized trial determines that topical ocular hypotensive medication delays or prevents the onset of primary open-angle glaucoma. *Arch. Ophthalmol.* **2002**, *120*, 701–713. [CrossRef]
5. Li, F.; Huang, W.; Zhang, X. Efficacy and safety of different regiments for primary open-angle glaucoma or ocular hypertension: A systemic review and network meta-analysis. *Acta Ophthalmol.* **2018**, *96*, e277–e284. [CrossRef] [PubMed]
6. Robin, A.L.; Covert, D. Does adjunctive glaucoma therapy affect adherence to the initial primary therapy? *Ophthalmology* **2005**, *112*, 863–868. [CrossRef]
7. Robin, A.L.; Novack, G.D.; Covert, D.W.; Crockett, R.S.; Marcic, T.S. Adherence in glaucoma: Objective measurements of once-daily and adjunctive medication use. *Am. J. Ophthalmol.* **2007**, *144*, 533–540. [CrossRef]
8. Higginbotham, E.J.; Hansen, J.; Davis, E.J.; Walt, J.G.; Guckian, A. Glaucoma medication persistence with a fixed combination versus multiple bottles. *Curr. Med Res. Opin.* **2009**, *25*, 2543–2547. [CrossRef]
9. Bangalore, S.; Kamalakkannan, G.; Parkar, S.; Messerli, F.H. Fixed-dose combinations improve medication compliance: A meta-analysis. *Am. J. Med.* **2007**, *120*, 713–719. [CrossRef]
10. Fechtner, R.D.; Myers, J.S.; Hubatsch, D.A.; Budenz, D.L.; DuBiner, H.B. Ocular hypotensive effects of fixed-combination brinzolamide/brimonidine adjunctive to a prostaglandin analog: A randomized clinical trial. *Eye* **2016**, *30*, 1343–1350. [CrossRef]
11. Feldman, R.M.; Katz, G.; McMenemy, M.; Hubatsch, D.A.; Realini, T. A randomized trial of fixed-dose combination brinzolamide 1%/brimonidine 0.2% as adjunctive therapy to travoprost 0.004. *Am. J. Ophthalmol.* **2016**, *165*, 188–197. [CrossRef]
12. Topouzis, F.; Goldberg, I.; Bell, K.; Tatham, A.J.; Ridolfi, A.; Hubatsch, D.; Nicolela, M.; Denis, P.; Lerner, S.F. Brinzolamide/brimonidine fixed-dose combination bid as an adjunct to a prostaglandin analog for open-angle glaucoma/ocular hypertension. *Eur. J. Ophthalmol.* **2021**, *31*, 103–111. [CrossRef] [PubMed]
13. Miyata, K.; Amano, S.; Sawa, M.; Nishida, T. A novel grading method for superficial punctate keratopathy magnitude and its correlation with corneal epithelial permeability. *Arch. Ophthalmol.* **2003**, *121*, 1537–1539. [CrossRef] [PubMed]
14. Bharmal, M.; Payne, K.; Atkinson, M.J.; Desrosiers, M.P.; Morisky, D.E.; Gemmen, E. Validation of an abbreviated Treatment Satisfaction Questionnaire for Medication (TSQM-9) among patients on antihypertensive medications. *Health Qual. Life Outcomes* **2009**, *7*, 36. [CrossRef] [PubMed]
15. Gandolfi, S.A.; Lim, J.; Sanseau, A.C.; Parra Restrepo, J.C.; Hamacher, T. Randomized trial of brinzolamide/brimonidine versus brinzolamide plus brimonidine for open-angle glaucoma or ocular hypertension. *Adv. Ther.* **2014**, *31*, 1213–1227. [CrossRef] [PubMed]
16. Steven, D.W.; Alaghband, P.; Lim, K.S. Preservatives in glaucoma medication. *Br. J. Ophthalmol.* **2018**, *102*, 1497–1503. [CrossRef]
17. Nakagawa, S.; Usui, T.; Yokoo, S.; Omichi, S.; Kimakura, M.; Mori, Y.; Miyata, K.; Aihara, M.; Amano, S.; Araie, M. Toxicity evaluation of antiglaucoma drugs using stratified human cultivated corneal epithelial sheets. *Investig. Ophthalmol. Vis. Sci.* **2012**, *53*, 5154–5160. [CrossRef]
18. Ingram, P.R.; Pitt, A.R.; Wilson, C.G.; Olejnik, O.; Spickett, C.M. A comparison of the effects of ocular preservatives on mammalian and microbial ATP and glutathione levels. *Free Radic. Res.* **2004**, *38*, 739–750. [CrossRef] [PubMed]
19. Meyer, T.; Funke, A.; Münch, C.; Kettemann, D.; Maier, A.; Walter, B.; Thomas, A.; Spittel, S. Real world experience of patients with amyotrophic lateral sclerosis (ALS) in the treatment of spasticity using tetrahydrocannabinol: Cannabidiol (THC:CBD). *BMC Neurol.* **2019**, *19*, 222. [CrossRef] [PubMed]
20. Contoli, M.; Rogliani, P.; Di Marco, F.; Braido, F.; Corsico, A.G.; Amici, C.A.; Piro, R.; Sarzani, R.; Lessi, P.; Scognamillo, C.; et al. Satisfaction with chronic obstructive pulmonary disease treatment: Results from a multicenter, observational study. *Ther. Adv. Respir. Dis.* **2019**, *13*, 175336661988128. [CrossRef] [PubMed]
21. Djafari, F.; Lesk, M.R.; Harasymowycz, P.J.; Desjardins, D.; Lachaine, J. Determinants of adherence to glaucoma medical therapy in a long-term patient population J. *Glaucoma* **2009**, *18*, 238–243. [CrossRef]
22. Rotchford, A.P.; Murphy, K.M. Compliance with timolol treatment in glaucoma. *Eye* **1998**, *12*, 234–236. [CrossRef]

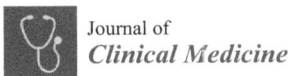

Article

Comparison of Treatment Outcomes of Selective Laser Trabeculoplasty for Primary Open-Angle Glaucoma and Pseudophakic Primary Angle-Closure Glaucoma Receiving Maximal Medical Therapy

Pei-Yao Chang [1,2,3,4,*], Jiun-Yi Wang [3,5], Jia-Kang Wang [1,2,4], Tzu-Lun Huang [1,4] and Yung-Ray Hsu [1,2,4]

1. Department of Ophthalmology, Far Eastern Memorial Hospital, Ban-Chiao, New Taipei City 220, Taiwan; jiakangw2158@gmail.com (J.-K.W.); huang.tzulum@gmail.com (T.-L.H.); scherzoray@gmail.com (Y.-R.H.)
2. Department of Medicine, National Taiwan University Hospital, Taipei City 100, Taiwan
3. Department of Healthcare Administration, Asia University, Taichung City 413, Taiwan; jjwang@asia.edu.tw
4. Department of Electrical Engineering, Yuan Ze University, Taoyuan City 320, Taiwan
5. Department of Medical Research, China Medical University Hospital, China Medical University, Taichung City 404, Taiwan
* Correspondence: peiyao@seed.net.tw; Tel.: +886-8966-7000

Citation: Chang, P.-Y.; Wang, J.-Y.; Wang, J.-K.; Huang, T.-L.; Hsu, Y.-R. Comparison of Treatment Outcomes of Selective Laser Trabeculoplasty for Primary Open-Angle Glaucoma and Pseudophakic Primary Angle-Closure Glaucoma Receiving Maximal Medical Therapy. *J. Clin. Med.* **2021**, *10*, 2853. https://doi.org/10.3390/jcm10132853

Academic Editor: Georgios Labiris

Received: 6 May 2021
Accepted: 25 June 2021
Published: 28 June 2021

Publisher's Note: MDPI stays neutral with regard to jurisdictional claims in published maps and institutional affiliations.

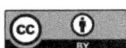

Copyright: © 2021 by the authors. Licensee MDPI, Basel, Switzerland. This article is an open access article distributed under the terms and conditions of the Creative Commons Attribution (CC BY) license (https://creativecommons.org/licenses/by/4.0/).

Abstract: Selective laser trabeculoplasty (SLT) is a useful treatment for intraocular pressure (IOP) control. However, there are only a few reports which compare the outcomes of SLT between primary open-angle glaucoma (POAG) and primary angle-closure glaucoma (PACG). We compared the efficacy of SLT for patients with PACG following phacoemulsification with POAG receiving maximal medical therapy (MMT). Consecutive glaucoma patients followed up for at least 1 year after SLT were retrospectively evaluated and IOP reductions at 6 months and 12 months were analyzed. Seventy-six patients were included in the analyses. The baseline IOPs in the POAG and PACG group were 18.5 ± 3.3 mmHg and 16.9 ± 2.5 mmHg, respectively, with 2.8 ± 0.9 and 2.7 ± 0.8 types of IOP lowering medication. The average IOP at the 6-month and 12-month follow-up after SLT was significantly decreased and comparable in both the POAG and PACG groups. For those with a low baseline IOP, the effect of SLT on IOP reduction at 12 months was significantly better in the PACG than in the POAG group ($p = 0.003$). IOP reduction at 6 and 12 months after SLT was significantly greater in those with a high baseline IOP than those with a low baseline IOP ($p < 0.0065$). In summary, the one-year efficacy of SLT was equivalent in POAG and pseudophakic PACG patients receiving MMT; however, SLT was more effective in eyes with PACG than eyes with POAG when focusing on those with a lower baseline IOP.

Keywords: selective laser trabeculoplasty; intraocular pressure; glaucoma

1. Introduction

Intraocular pressure (IOP) control is currently the only well-established treatment for glaucoma to slow or prevent further visual field progression. Selective laser trabeculoplasty (SLT) is an efficient IOP-lowering treatment for primary open angle glaucoma (POAG) and ocular hypertension [1,2]. Studies have proved that SLT can be used as an initial treatment or in combination with IOP-lowing drugs when the topical medications could not obtain satisfactory therapeutic effects in patients with POAG [1,3–5].

Primary angle closure glaucoma (PACG) is common in Asia. Laser peripheral iridotomy (LPI) is the current first-line treatment in the management of PACG and argon laser peripheral iridoplasty has also been shown to dramatically lower the IOP and open up the closed angles [6]. However, medical therapy is often required after LPI for IOP control [7]. Studies have reported that SLT is a safe and cost-effective modality for reducing IOP in post LPI PACG [8–10]. A multicenter randomized trial demonstrated the comparable effect in PACG patients between SLT treatment and topical prostaglandin analog usage [8]. Therefore, SLT is also a potential therapeutic option in patients with PACG.

Cataract and glaucoma frequently coexist in elderly PACG patients. Numerous studies have demonstrated a modest reduction in IOP and angle widening following cataract surgery in patients with PACG [11–13]. However, trabecular damage may result in IOP elevation even after opening of the anterior chamber angles by cataract surgery in eyes with long-standing iridotrabecular apposition [14]. Patients with severe glaucomatous optic neuropathy and IOP fluctuation even following cataract surgery may require additional IOP-lowering treatment, including long-term glaucoma medications or even surgical intervention. Tham et al. reported both phacoemulsification and trabeculectomy were effective in reducing IOP in chronic angle closure glaucoma, but 19% of patients from the phacoemulsification arm did eventually require trabeculectomy in the 2-year follow-up period [15]. SLT has fewer complications, as compared to surgery, whether trabeculectomy or even minimally invasive glaucoma surgery [8,15]. SLT addresses the issue of compliance associated with topical medications and offers a treatment option in a select group of patients with PACG whose angle has been widened after lens removal but still having unsatisfactory IOP control.

Limited studies have been evaluated regarding SLT as an adjunctive treatment modality for PACG. Therefore, we performed a retrospective study in a mid-term follow-up of one year to observe the outcomes of SLT in patients with PACG following phacoemulsification and intraocular lens implantation (PEA + IOL) and compared the outcomes of SLT in patients with POAG.

2. Materials and Methods

This was a retrospective chart review study, which included patients who had SLT performed by one glaucoma specialist (PYC) between January 2015 and December 2018. The study protocol was approved by the Ethics Committee of our institution (No.: 109108-E) and the study adhered to the tenets of the Declaration of Helsinki. Baseline demographic data such as age, gender, IOP, visual field mean deviation, total laser power, types of glaucoma, history of ocular surgery, and the number of glaucoma medications were collected from medical charts.

The IOP usually significantly decreases in angle closure glaucoma patients following cataract surgery [11–13]. Most PACG patients choose conservative treatments (topical medications) following PEA+IOL to control IOP, and SLT was the most considered treatment option when the maximal medical therapy (MMT) failed in these circumstances in our hospital. Moreover, we performed SLT mostly as an adjunct treatment with unsatisfactory IOP control with visual field progression in patients with POAG. Therefore, the current study included patients with POAG or PACG with unsatisfactory IOP control with visual field progression even receiving MMT or patients without visual field progression but intolerability to MMT. The degree of SLT treatment was variable in PACG patients, depending on extent of remaining peripheral anterior synechia (PAS) following phacoemulsification. Because we routinely performed 270° SLT treatment in open angle glaucoma, we included PACG patients only when they had at least 270° of trabecular meshwork (TM) visible by gonioscopy without corneal indentation or manipulation after uncomplicated phacoemulsification.

Exclusion criteria were secondary glaucoma, previous ophthalmic surgery, except for uncomplicated cataract surgery, and previous ophthalmic laser, except LPI. However, LPI and uncomplicated phacoemulsification must be performed at least 12 months prior to SLT treatment. We excluded any other form of open angle glaucoma other than POAG, such as pigmentary glaucoma or pseudoexfoliation glaucoma. Filtering surgery instead of SLT was usually considered in such cases in our routine practice.

SLT was performed using the Selecta Duet laser (Lumenis, Dreieich, Germany) (frequency doubled, Q-switched Nd: YAG 532 nm, 3-ns pulse, spot size 400 μm). The initial power setting was between 0.6 and 0.8 mJ and the energy was increased or decreased by

0.1 mJ until a small bubble formation appeared for the remaining treatment. The procedure was then completed for 270°, avoiding areas of PAS and areas with limited visibility of the TM. A drop of brimonidine 0.2% was administered after laser therapy. IOP was measured 1 h after the procedure and patients who experienced a postoperative elevation of >5 mm Hg received oral carbonic anhydrase inhibitors.

Patients did not receive any topical anti-inflammatory medications and maintained the same preoperative IOP lowering drugs before the next visit. The amount of glaucoma medications prescribed in the postoperative period was decided according to the IOP level and glaucoma severity. Postoperative IOP data were collected at the 3-, 6-, 9- and 12-month visits with the noncontact computerized tonometer (CT-80, Topcon, Tokyo, Japan).

Statistical Analysis

Statistical analysis was performed using the SPSS software (v.22.0; IBM Corp, Armonk, NY, USA). Descriptive statistics such as the number and percentage for categorical data and the mean ± standard deviation for continuous data were used to present data distributions. Chi-squared test and the two-sample t test were respectively used to compare sample proportions and sample means of the two groups of POAG and PACG. The amount of ocular hypotensive drugs used before and after SLT was compared. IOP reductions from the baseline to the follow-up time-points were calculated and tested, based on paired t-test. Nonparametric methods such as Mann–Whitney U test and Wilcoxon signed-rank test were also conducted for a double check, due to the small to moderate sample size in the study. Considering that there were 5 and 9 missing IOP in the POAG group and 2 and 3 missing IOP in the PACG group for 6- and 12-month follow-up, respectively, the generalized estimating equations (GEE) analysis was implemented for repeated measures. It was used to evaluate whether the IOP reduction effect (at the time-points of 6 and 12 months) was different between groups, either open and closed type, high baseline IOP (IOP $\geq$ 17 mmHg) and low baseline IOP (IOP < 17 mmHg) group, or better VF (MD) and worse VF group. In each GEE model, age, sex, baseline IOP, and VF were included as control variables when appropriate, and the interaction terms of time and group were also included. A significance of an interaction in the model implies that the effect was different between groups. The significance level of all analyses was set at 0.05, except for comparisons of IOP changes between POAG and PACG patients for overall and subgroups, which was set at 0.0065 (=0.05/8) due to Bonferroni correction for multiple testing.

3. Results

3.1. Demographics of the Participants

Baseline characteristics, clinical parameters and topical medications of the study participants were displayed in Table 1. There were 53 participants with POAG and 23 with PACG included in the analyses. The mean age (51.7 ± 10.9 vs. 66.3 ± 10.2 years old) and percentages of male (32.1% vs. 60.9%) were both significantly different between the groups of POAG and PACG. Significantly worse VF, lower baseline IOP and higher presence of PAS in the PACG group were observed. However, there was no significant difference in the indications for SLT between the two groups. Table 2 shows that the number of bottles and the types of ocular hypotensive drugs, as well as the proportion of each of the four types of drugs, had no significant difference after SLT in either group.

Table 1. Baseline characteristics of SLT treated eyes in PACG and POAG groups.

	POAG	PACG	p-Value [a]
Number of patients	53	23	
Age (years)	51.7 ± 10.9	66.3 ± 10.2	<0.001
Male gender	17 (32.1%)	14 (60.9%)	0.024
Mean deviation (dB)	−11.3 ± 7.3	−16.3 ± 7.7	0.011
IOP (mmHg)	18.5 ± 3.3	16.9 ± 2.5	0.026
Central corneal thickness (μm)	565.9 ± 31.1	555.6 ± 33.6	0.224
Circumpapillary retinal nerve fiber layer (μm)	69.3 ± 12.7	65.0 ± 9.6	0.129
Pseudophakic	4 (7.5%)	23 (100%)	<0.001
Presence of peripheral anterior synechia	0 (0%)	4 (17.4%)	0.007
Indication for SLT			1.000
Uncontrolled IOP	45 (84.9%)	20 (87.0%)	
Intolerability to Topical medication	8 (15.1%)	3 (13.0%)	
Topical medication			
Bottle	2.1 ± 0.6	2.1 ± 0.5	0.851
Type	2.8 ± 0.9	2.7 ± 0.8	0.530
A-agonist	24 (45.3%)	15 (65.2%)	0.138
β-blocker	45 (84.9%)	16 (69.6%)	0.208
Prostaglandin analog	47 (88.7%)	20 (87.0%)	1.000
Carbonic anhydrase inhibitor	34 (64.2%)	11 (47.8%)	0.211

[a] p-values of two-sample t test. The results of testing for continuous data based on Mann–Whitney U test were the same and thus not shown here.

Table 2. Comparisons of the amount of ocular hypotensive drugs before and one year after SLT.

	Before SLT		After SLT		
	Mean ± SD	(%)	Mean ± SD	(%)	p-Value [a]
POAG					
Bottle	2.1 ± 0.6		2.2 ± 0.6		0.419
Type	2.8 ± 0.9		2.9 ± 0.9		0.444
A-agonist		45.3%		45.3%	1.000
β-blocker		84.9%		84.9%	1.000
Prostaglandin analog		88.7%		90.6%	1.000
Carbonic anhydrase inhibitor		64.2%		67.9%	0.727
PACG					
Bottle	2.1 ± 0.5		2.1 ± 0.6		1.000
Type	2.7 ± 0.8		2.7 ± 1.0		0.665
A-agonist		65.2%		69.6%	0.629
β-blocker		69.6%		73.9%	1.000
Prostaglandin analog		87.0%		95.7%	0.500
Carbonic anhydrase inhibitor		47.8%		34.8%	0.250

[a] p-values of paired t test. The results of testing for continuous data based on Wilcoxon signed-rank test were the same and thus not shown here.

3.2. IOP Change

The IOP change is displayed in Table 3. The average IOP at the 6-month and 12-month follow-up after SLT had significantly decreased in both POAG and PACG group. When we further divided patients into a high baseline IOP (IOP ≥ 17 mmHg) and a low baseline IOP (IOP < 17 mmHg) group, the average IOP decreased significantly for those with a high baseline IOP in both the POAG and PACG group. For those with a low baseline IOP, it had decreased significantly at the 12-month follow-up after SLT only in the PACG group.

Table 3. IOP values and the reduction before and after SLT of all cases and subgroups of higher and lower IOP. (High IOP: baseline IOP ≥ 17 mmHg; low IOP: baseline IOP < 17 mmHg.).

Group Time-Point	n	IOP (Mean ± SD)	IOP Reduction (Mean ± SD)	IOP Reduction Percentage (%)	p-Value [a]
POAG (all cases)					
Baseline	53	18.5 ± 3.3			
6 months	48	15.6 ± 3.2	2.9 ± 3.4	15.5%	<0.001
12 months	44	16.1 ± 3.5	2.7 ± 3.1	13.0%	<0.001
POAG (high IOP)					
Baseline	36	20.2 ± 2.6			
6 months	32	16.3 ± 3.0	3.9 ± 3.2	19.1%	<0.001
12 months	31	16.7 ± 3.7	3.6 ± 3.1	16.9%	<0.001
POAG (low IOP)					
Baseline	17	15.0 ± 1.1			
6 months	16	14.2 ± 3.2	0.8 ± 2.7	4.9%	0.250
12 months	13	14.5 ± 2.3	0.5 ± 1.6	3.2%	0.261
PACG (all cases)					
Baseline	23	16.9 ± 2.5			
6 months	21	14.8 ± 2.7	2.1 ± 3.1	12.6%	0.005
12 months	20	13.3 ± 2.2	3.3 ± 1.9	21.5%	<0.001
PACG (high IOP)					
Baseline	14	18.5 ± 1.9			
6 months	12	15.4 ± 2.6	3.3 ± 2.9	16.5%	0.002
12 months	11	14.3 ± 2.1	4.1 ± 2.0	22.6%	<0.001
PACG (low IOP)					
Baseline	9	14.5 ± 1.0			
6 months	9	13.9 ± 2.7	0.6 ± 2.7	3.1%	0.545
12 months	9	12.0 ± 1.6	2.5 ± 1.5	13.3%	<0.001

[a] p-values of paired t test. The results of testing based on Wilcoxon signed-rank test were the same and thus not shown.

Table 4 summarizes the results of the interaction terms from the GEE analyses. It demonstrated that the interactions of time and the types of glaucoma were not significant ($p = 0.327$ and 0.135 at 6 and 12 months). For those with low baseline IOP, the effects on IOP reduction at 12 months after SLT were significantly better in the PACG than in the POAG group ($p = 0.003$). In patients with POAG, the IOP reduction at both 6 and 12 months after SLT was significantly more in the high baseline IOP group than the low baseline IOP group, while the effects on reducing IOP at both 6 and 12 months after SLT had no significant difference between the better and worse VF group.

None of the eyes experienced IOP elevation of >10 mm Hg, whereas 2 (3.8%) eyes with POAG had 5 mm Hg IOP elevation within 1 h of SLT. No permanent adverse effects of SLT were noted in any of the patients.

Table 4. Comparisons of IOP changes between POAG and PACG patients for overall and subgroups (A) and between patients with high and low VF or higher and lower baseline IOP for subgroups of POAG and PACG (B), based on the GEE analysis. All models included the main effects of the interaction terms and were adjusted for age, sex, pre IOP group, and VF group where appropriate.

Model		95%CI		
Subgroup Interaction Term	B	Lower Limit	Upper Limit	p-Value
(A)				
All patients				
(PACG vs. POAG) and (6th month vs. baseline)	0.78	−0.78	2.35	0.327
(PACG vs. POAG) and (12th month vs. baseline)	−0.98	−2.26	0.30	0.135
1. Baseline IOP ≥ 17 mmHg				
(PACG vs. POAG) and (6th month vs. baseline)	0.71	−1.17	2.59	0.459
(PACG vs. POAG) and (12th month vs. baseline)	−0.78	−2.53	0.97	0.381
2. Baseline IOP < 17 mmHg				
(PACG vs. POAG) and (6th month vs. baseline)	0.23	−1.87	2.33	0.828
(PACG vs. POAG) and (12th month vs. baseline)	−1.85	−3.07	−0.63	0.003
3. Visual field defect ≥ 12 dB				
(PACG vs. POAG) and (6th month vs. baseline)	0.76	−1.42	2.94	0.495
(PACG vs. POAG) and (12th month vs. baseline)	−1.31	−3.00	0.39	0.130
4. Visual field defect < 12 dB				
(PACG vs. POAG) and (6th month vs. baseline)	0.46	−1.49	2.41	0.644
(PACG vs. POAG) and (12th month vs. baseline)	−0.68	−2.68	1.33	0.509
(B)				
1. POAG				
(VF: higher vs. lower) and (6th month vs. baseline)	0.16	−1.73	2.06	0.867
(VF: higher vs. lower) and (12th month vs. baseline)	0.54	−1.21	2.29	0.545
2. PACG				
(VF: higher vs. lower) and (6th month vs. baseline)	0.41	−1.91	2.73	0.730
(VF: higher vs. lower) and (12th month vs. baseline)	−0.16	−1.89	1.56	0.852
3. POAG				
(pre IOP: higher vs. lower) and (6th month vs. baseline)	−3.03	−4.72	−1.35	<0.001
(pre IOP: higher vs. lower) and (12th month vs. baseline)	−2.94	−4.24	−1.63	<0.001
4. PACG				
(pre IOP: higher vs. lower) and (6th month vs. baseline)	−2.49	−4.78	−0.20	0.033
(pre IOP: higher vs. lower) and (12th month vs. baseline)	−1.71	−3.32	−0.10	0.038

4. Discussion

Studies comparing the effectiveness of SLT in PACG and POAG are inconclusive and the data regarding the efficacy in PACG eyes is rather limited. We have summarized the efficacy of SLT in patients with PACG in Table 5. Most studies reporting the efficacy of SLT in PACG patients did not focus on PACG patients following cataract surgery [8–10,16]; while this is the first study which evaluated PACG patients only following PEA+IOL. Natalia IK [16] reported there was no significant difference in the one-year efficacy of SLT between POAG and PACG, which was similar to our findings when we did not divide patients into high and low IOP group. However, they excluded patients who underwent phacoemulsification and their baseline IOP prior to SLT was 23.18 ± 3.53 mmHg in PACG and 22.23 ± 2.99 mmHg in POAG, which was higher than that in our study population. Ali Aljasim et al. [8] showed that the success rate of SLT in PACG was better than that in

POAG, although it did not reach a significant level. One thing in their study that needs to be addressed was that the percentage of 360-degree of SLT application and the laser energy was significantly higher in their POAG group, while the success rate was 84% in the PACG and 79% in the POAG group. Our study highlighted SLT had better efficacy in patients with PACG compared to POAG, but was only found in patients with IOP less than 17 mmHg. We found in the group of PACG with IOP less than 17 mmHg, IOP was 14.5 ± 1.0 mmHg at baseline and 12.0 ± 1.6 mmHg 1 year after SLT treatment, the IOP reduction percentage (13.3%) in the PACG group was significantly more than that in POAG group (3.2%).

Table 5. Summary of efficacy of SLT in patients with primary angle-closure glaucoma.

Paper	Design	Number of Eyes	Postoperative Follow-up	Definition of Success	Success Rate	Average IOP Reduction
Ali Aljasim et al. [8] (2016)	Retrospective case–control study	$n = 59$ (PAC/PACG), $n = 59$ (POAG)	PAC/PACG: 6–20 months POAG: 6–17 months	IOP reduction ≥ 20% without further medical or surgical intervention or a reduction in the number of glaucoma medications by ≥1 while maintaining the target IOP	PAC/PACG: 84.7%, POAG: 79.6% $p = 0.47$	IOP reduction in patients with uncontrolled IOP: 38% (PAC/PACG) vs. 32.7% (POAG), $p = 0.08$
Narayanaswamy et al. [9] (2015)	Randomized clinical trial	$n = 50$ (SLT), $n = 50$ (PGA)	6 months	Complete success: IOP lower than 21 mmHg without any additional IOP-lowering medications Qualified success: IOP lower than 21 mmHg who required IOP lowering medication	Complete success: 60% (SLT) vs. 84% (PGA), $p = 0.008$ Qualified success: 18% (SLT) vs. 6% (PGA), $p = 0.06$	16.9% (SLT) vs. 18.5% (PGA) $p = 0.52$
Raj et al. [10] (2018)	Prospective cross-sectional study	$n = 34$ (23 PAC and 11 PACG)	1 year	N/A	N/A	3 month: 19.61% 6 month: 22.43% 1 year: 28.7%
Kurysheva et al. [16] (2018)	Retrospective case–control study	$n = 68$ (PACG), $n = 74$ (POAG)	PACG/PACG: 6.94 ± 1.92 years POAG: 6.34 ± 1.94 years	20% IOP reduction with topical hypotensive medications without any hypotensive intervention (repeated SLT, antiglaucoma surgery, phacoemulsification of cataracts)	PACG vs. POAG 2 years: 66% vs. 62% 3 years: 62% vs. 54% 4 years: 44% vs. 38% 5 years: 42% vs. 36% 6 years: 6% vs. 4% $p = 0.24$	At 6 years, reduction in mean baseline IOP from 23.57 ± 2.30 to 18.77 ± 2.25 (PACG) and from 22.45 ± 1.46 to 18.86 ± 2.09 (POAG)
Kurysheva et al. [17] (2019)	Prospective longitudinal study	$n = 60$ (PACG), $n = 64$ (POAG)	PACG: 6.75 ± 1.83 years POAG: 6.22 ± 1.54 years	20% IOP reduction with topical hypotensive medications without any hypotensive intervention (repeated SLT, antiglaucoma surgery, and phacoemulsification).	PACG vs. POAG 1 year: 89% vs. 90% 6 year: 34% vs. 36%	N/A [a]

[a] N/A: not applicable (IOP reduction percentage was not shown in this study).

The injuries to the conventional aqueous outflow system induced by angle closure are variable and depend on various anatomic factors [6]. The mechanisms of angle closure can be divided into three groups: (i) appositional, leading to pretrabecular obstruction without TM injury; (ii) appositional with TM obstruction associated with structural and functional modifications due to chronic contact; (iii) synechial, accompanied by permanent adherence [18]. We excluded angle closure patients who had a history of acute attack and included those only with visible TM over 270°. It is impossible to differentiate type (i) and (ii) by clinical examinations, but patients in the group of PACG with IOP less than 17 mmHg after PEA + IOL would probably be those who had less TM injury induced by angle closure. Moreover, TM height was reported to be shorter in PACG patients compared to POAG patients [19]. Since the spot size and duration of SLT was fixed, the laser energy might be more concentrated in a smaller tissue. As for the reason why SLT was more effective in the low IOP group in PACG only at the 1-year follow-up but not at the 6-month follow-up was unclear. However, it was reported that Raj et al. [10] found the percentage of eyes without medication achieving IOP in the level of 12–15 mmHg was 9% at 6 months but increased to 35.7% at the 1-year follow-up in PACG patients.

The published literature reporting the outcomes of SLT varies widely with IOP reductions ranging from 6.9% up to 35.9% of baseline IOP [1–5,8–10,20–24]. Primary SLT achieved IOP reductions of 29.7% in OHT eyes and 26.1% in OAG eyes [1]. IOP reduction varied widely depending on different study populations, baseline IOP and the degree of laser application. The IOP reduction percentage in the POAG group was relatively low in our study, which was 15.5% at the 6-month and 13% at the 12-month follow-up. Our baseline IOPs (18.5 ± 3.3 mmHg in POAG group and 16.9 ± 2.5 mmHg in PACG group) were lower compared with those in previous studies. Most of the evidence pointed at a higher success rate and/or greater IOP reduction in eyes with a higher baseline IOP [3,16,19,21], and we also had the same findings in both groups, although it only reached the significant level in the POAG group. SLT achieved more than 20% IOP reduction in 95% of eyes in medically controlled glaucoma patients with a 1.5 baseline number of medications [4]. However, greater usage of hypotensive eye drops before SLT was associated with a higher risk of failure for both POAG and PACG patients [16]. In our study, patients used MMT with approximately 2.1 bottles, 2.7 types of hypotensive eye drops before SLT treatment. The one-year efficacy of SLT was very limited in patients under MMT with only 14.2% of patients reaching IOP reduction > 20% [5], which was in agreement with our findings. The amount of ocular hypotensive drugs before and after SLT was not significantly different in this study because we performed SLT mainly as an adjunctive therapy. We did not reduce the current medications despite successful SLT since most of the patients in this study had moderate to severe glaucoma.

In some respects, the baseline characteristics were not similar between the two groups. All of the PACG patients while only 7.5% of the POAG patients were pseudophakic in our cohort. However, the IOP-lowering effect of SLT treatment was reported to be comparable between pseudophakic and phakic eyes in prospective [19] and retrospective studies [23,24]. Moreover, the baseline VF defect was significantly more and the baseline IOP was significantly less in our PACG group than that in our POAG group, which was quite reasonable that lower target IOP was usually set in severer patients. In our hospital, we were more conservative when considering SLT as a supplementary treatment in PACG patients who had received cataract surgery based on the following two reasons: first, good outcomes in terms of IOP control have been found following lens extraction for PACG [10]. Numerous studies even suggest PEA+IOL is a feasible option for IOP control in PACG [13]. Second, slower VF progression rate in PACG compared to high tension glaucoma and normal tension glaucoma when baseline severity was matched [25]. Therefore, if the IOP and VF were stable after PEA+IOL, SLT would not be suggested unless topical antiglaucoma medication was not tolerable.

Our study has its limitations including retrospective design, lack of information of angle pigmentation, a small sample size and a limited follow-up period. Moreover, the baseline demographics were different between the two groups. However, we adjusted gender, age and even baseline IOP in relevant analyses, and we included only those PACG patients with at least 270° of TM visible by gonioscopy, therefore the extent of laser application was the same in the two groups. Lastly, Goldman applanation tonometer was the gold standard of IOP measurement, but mostly we used it in prospective glaucoma studies. Due to the retrospective design, a noncontact tonometer was used in this study. In summary, the one-year efficacy of SLT was equivalent in POAG and PACG patients receiving MMT; however, SLT was more effective in eyes with PACG than eyes with POAG when focusing on those with a lower baseline IOP. Although our sample size is fairly small to reach definitive conclusions, it is worthy of note that these groups of patients may still benefit from SLT. Our results suggest clinicians may consider SLT as a supplementary treatment in eyes with PACG after PEA+IOL even when the IOP is lower than 17 mmHg. Further studies would be required to explore the long-term effect of SLT in PACG patients with low IOP following cataract surgery.

5. Conclusions

In summary, the one-year efficacy of SLT was equivalent in POAG and PACG patients receiving MMT; however, SLT was more effective in eyes with PACG than eyes with POAG when focusing on those with a lower baseline IOP.

Author Contributions: Conceptualization, P.-Y.C. and J.-Y.W.; methodology, J.-Y.W.; software, Y.-R.H.; validation, J.-Y.W., Y.-R.H.; formal analysis, J.-Y.W.; investigation, P.-Y.C., J.-Y.W., Y.-R.H., T.-L.H. and J.-K.W.; resources, P.-Y.C.; data curation, P.-Y.C.; writing—original draft preparation, P.-Y.C.; writing—review and editing, P.-Y.C. and J.-Y.W.; visualization, T.-L.H.; supervision, J.-K.W.; project administration, J.-K.W.; funding acquisition, P.-Y.C. All authors have read and agreed to the published version of the manuscript.

Funding: This project was supported by a grant obtained from the Far Eastern Memorial Hospital (FEMH-2021-C049).

Institutional Review Board Statement: The study was approved by the institutional review board of the Far Eastern Memorial Hospital, Taipei, Taiwan (No.109108-E), which waived the requirement for informed consent from participants and allowed access to the follow-up clinical records. It was conducted in accordance with the requirements of the Declaration of Helsinki.

Informed Consent Statement: Patient consent was waived due to the retrospective type of this study, and the IRB waived the requirement for obtaining informed consent.

Data Availability Statement: Data will not be shared because the authors are performing other analyses that have not yet been published.

Conflicts of Interest: The authors declare no conflict of interest.

References

1. Garg, A.; Vickerstaff, V.; Nathwani, N.; Garway-Heath, D.; Konstantakopoulou, E.; Ambler, G.; Bunce, C.; Wormald, R.; Barton, K.; Gazzard, G. Laser in ocular hypertension trial study, primary selective laser trabeculoplasty for open-angle glaucoma and ocular hypertension: Clinical outcomes, predictors of success, and safety from the laser in glaucoma and ocular hypertension trial. *Ophthalmology* **2019**, *126*, 1238–1248. [CrossRef]
2. Gazzard, G.; Konstantakopoulou, E.; Garway-Heath, D.; Garg, A.; Vickerstaff, V.; Hunter, R.; Ambler, G.; Bunce, C.; Wormald, R.; Nathwani, N. Selective laser trabeculoplasty versus eye drops for first-line treatment of ocular hypertension and glaucoma (LiGHT): A multicentre randomised controlled trial. *Lancet* **2019**, *393*, 1505–1516. [CrossRef]
3. Lee, J.W.; Wong, M.O.; Liu, C.C.; Lai, J.S. Optimal selective laser trabeculoplasty energy for maximal intraocular pressure reduction in open-angle glaucoma. *J. Glaucoma* **2015**, *24*, e128–e131. [CrossRef] [PubMed]
4. De Keyser, M.; De Belder, M.; De Belder, J.; De Groot, V. Selective laser trabeculoplasty as replacement therapy in medically controlled glaucoma patients. *Acta Ophthalmol.* **2018**, *96*, e577–e581. [CrossRef] [PubMed]
5. Miki, A.; Kawashima, R.; Usui, S.; Matsushita, K.; Nishida, K. Treatment outcomes and prognostic factors of selective laser trabeculoplasty for open-angle glaucoma receiving maximal-tolerable medical therapy. *J. Glaucoma* **2016**, *25*, 785–789. [CrossRef] [PubMed]
6. Sun, X.; Dai, Y.; Chen, Y.; Yu, D.Y.; Cringle, S.J.; Chen, J.; Kong, X.; Wang, X.; Jiang, C. Primary angle closure glaucoma: What we know and what we don't know. *Prog. Retin. Eye Res.* **2017**, *57*, 26–45. [CrossRef]

7. Peng, P.H.; Nguyen, H.; Lin, H.S.; Nguyen, N.; Lin, S. Long-term outcomes of laser iridotomy in Vietnamese patients with primary angle closure. *Br. J. Ophthalmol.* **2011**, *95*, 1207–1211. [CrossRef] [PubMed]
8. Aljasim, L.A.; Owaidhah, O.; Edward, D.P. Selective laser trabeculoplasty in primary angle-closure glaucoma after laser peripheral iridotomy: A case–control study. *J. Glaucoma* **2016**, *25*, e253–e258. [CrossRef] [PubMed]
9. Narayanaswamy, A.; Leung, C.K.; Istiantoro, D.V.; Perera, S.A.; Ho, C.L.; Nongpiur, M.E.; Baskaran, M.; Htoon, H.M.; Wong, T.T.; Goh, D.; et al. Efficacy of selective laser trabeculoplasty in primary angle-closure glaucoma: A randomized clinical trial. *JAMA Ophthalmol.* **2015**, *133*, 206–212. [CrossRef] [PubMed]
10. Raj, S.; Tigari, B.; Faisal, T.T.; Gautam, N.; Kaushik, S.; Ichhpujani, P.; Pandav, S.S.; Ram, J. Efficacy of selective laser trabeculoplasty in primary angle closure disease. *Eye* **2018**, *32*, 1710–1716. [CrossRef]
11. Trikha, S.; Perera, S.A.; Husain, R.; Aung, T. The role of lens extraction in the current management of primary angle-closure glaucoma. *Curr. Opin. Ophthalmol.* **2015**, *26*, 128–234. [CrossRef]
12. Lai, J.S.; Tham, C.C.; Chan, J.C. The clinical outcomes of cataract extraction by phacoemulsification in eyes with primary angle-closure glaucoma (PACG) and co-existing cataract: A prospective case series. *J. Glaucoma* **2006**, *15*, 47–52. [CrossRef] [PubMed]
13. Azuara-Blanco, A.; Burr, J.; Ramsay, C.; Cooper, D.; Foster, P.J.; Friedman, D.S.; Scotland, G.; Javanbakht, M.; Cochrane, C.; Norrie, J. Effectiveness of early lens extraction for the treatment of primary angle-closure glaucoma (EAGLE): A randomised controlled trial. *Lancet* **2016**, *388*, 1389–1397. [CrossRef]
14. Tham, C.C.; Kwong, Y.Y.; Leung, D.Y.; Lam, S.W.; Li, F.C.; Chiu, T.Y.; Chan, J.C.; Chan, C.H.; Poon, A.S.; Yick, D.W.; et al. Phacoemulsification versus combined phacotrabeculectomy in medically controlled chronic angle closure glaucoma with cataract. *Ophthalmology* **2008**, *115*, 2167–2173. [CrossRef] [PubMed]
15. Tham, C.C.; Kwong, Y.Y.; Baig, N.; Leung, D.Y.; Li, F.C.; Lam, D.S. Phacoemulsification versus trabeculectomy in medically uncontrolled chronic angle-closure glaucoma without cataract. *Ophthalmology* **2013**, *120*, 62–67. [CrossRef]
16. Kurysheva, N.I.; Lepeshkina, L.V.; Shatalova, E.O. Predictors of outcome in selective laser trabeculoplasty: A long-term observation study in primary angle-closure glaucoma after laser peripheral iridotomy compared with primary open-angle glaucoma. *J. Glaucoma* **2018**, *27*, 880–886. [CrossRef] [PubMed]
17. Kurysheva, N.I.; Lepeshkina, L.V. Selective laser trabeculoplasty protects glaucoma progression in the initial primary open-angle glaucoma and angle-closure glaucoma after laser peripheral iridotomy in the long term. *BioMed Res. Int* **2019**, *2019*, 4519412. [CrossRef] [PubMed]
18. Matos, A.G.; Asrani, S.G.; Paula, J.S. Feasibility of laser trabeculoplasty in angle closure glaucoma: A review of favourable histopathological findings in narrow angles. *Clin. Exp. Ophthalmol.* **2017**, *45*, 632–639. [CrossRef] [PubMed]
19. Masis, M.; Chen, R.; Porco, T.; Lin, S.C. Trabecular meshwork height in primary open-angle glaucoma versus primary angle-closure glaucoma. *Am. J. Ophthalmol.* **2017**, *183*, 42–47. [CrossRef]
20. Wong, M.O.; Lee, J.W.; Choy, B.N.; Chan, J.C.; Lai, J.S. Systematic review and meta-analysis on the efficacy of selective laser trabeculoplasty in open-angle glaucoma. *Surv. Ophthalmol.* **2015**, *60*, 36–50. [CrossRef] [PubMed]
21. Chun, M.; Gracitelli, C.P.; Lopes, F.S.; Biteli, L.G.; Ushida, M.; Prata, T.S. Selective laser trabeculoplasty for early glaucoma: Analysis of success predictors and adjusted laser outcomes based on the untreated fellow eye. *BMC Ophthalmol.* **2016**, *16*, 206. [CrossRef] [PubMed]
22. De Keyser, M.; De Belder, M.; De Groot, V. Selective laser trabeculoplasty in pseudophakic and phakic eyes: A prospective study. *Int. J. Ophthalmol.* **2017**, *10*, 593–598. [PubMed]
23. Kalbag, N.; Patel, S.; Khouri, A.; Berezina, T.; Fechtner, R.; Cohen, A. Selective laser trabeculoplasty in the treatment of glaucoma in phakic versus pseudophakic patients. *Investig. Ophthalmol. Vis. Sci.* **2013**, *54*, 1862.
24. Seymenoglu, G.; Baser, E.F. Efficacy of selective laser trabeculoplasty in phakic and pseudophakic eyes. *J. Glaucoma* **2015**, *24*, 105–110. [CrossRef] [PubMed]
25. Ganeshrao, S.B.; Senthil, S.; Choudhari, N.; Durgam, S.S.; Garudadri, C.S. Comparison of visual field progression rates among the high tension glaucoma, primary angle closure glaucoma, and normal tension glaucoma. *Investig. Ophthalmol. Vis. Sci.* **2019**, *60*, 889–900. [CrossRef]

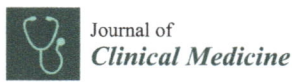

Article

Early Experience with the New XEN63 Implant in Primary Open-Angle Glaucoma Patients: Clinical Outcomes

Antonio Maria Fea [1,*], Martina Menchini [2], Alessandro Rossi [1], Chiara Posarelli [2], Lorenza Malinverni [1] and Michele Figus [2]

1. Struttura Complessa Oculistica, Città Della Salute e Della Scienza di Torino, Dipartimento di Scienze Chirurgiche-Università Degli Studi di Torino, 10126 Torino, Italy; alessandro.rossi012309@gmail.com (A.R.); lorenza.malinverni@unito.it (L.M.)
2. Department of Surgical, Medical and Molecular Pathology and Critical Care Medicine, University of Pisa, 56126 Pisa, Italy; martina.mmenchini@gmail.com (M.M.); chiara.posarelli@med.unipi.it (C.P.); michele.figus@unipi.it (M.F.)
* Correspondence: antoniomfea@gmail.com; Tel.: +39-349-560-1674

Abstract: The new XEN63 implant is a minimally invasive glaucoma surgery device with limited experience in real life. This retrospective study included open-angle glaucoma patients who underwent XEN63 implant, either alone or in combination with cataract surgery. Primary endpoints were the intraocular pressure (IOP) at month 3 and the incidence of serious adverse events. Twenty-three eyes of 23 patients were included. Mean age was 67.8 ± 15.3 years and 15 (65.2%) were women. Mean IOP was significantly lowered from 27.0 ± 7.8 mmHg at baseline to 12.2 ± 3.4 mmHg at month 3 ($p < 0.0001$). Mean IOP lowering was $40.8 \pm 23.5\%$, with 14 (60.9%) and 16 (69.6%) eyes achieving an IOP lowering $\geq 30\%$ and $\geq 20\%$ without hypotensive medication, respectively. The number of hypotensive medications (NHM) was significantly reduced from 2.27 ± 0.94 drugs at baseline to 0.09 ± 0.42 drugs at month 3, $p < 0.0001$. Four (17.4%) eyes had hypotony (IOP ≤ 6 mmHg) at postoperative day one, which was successfully resolved without sequelae. Four (17.4%) eyes had choroidal detachment (3 at day 7 and 1 at day 15), which was successfully resolved with medical treatment, at the month 1 visit. Three (13.0%) eyes required needling (mean time for needling 35.6 ± 9.7 days). XEN63 significantly lowered IOP and reduced the NHM, with a good short-term safety profile.

Keywords: glaucoma; open-angle glaucoma; XEN; minimally invasive glaucoma surgery; intraocular pressure; glaucoma surgery

Citation: Fea, A.M.; Menchini, M.; Rossi, A.; Posarelli, C.; Malinverni, L.; Figus, M. Early Experience with the New XEN63 Implant in Primary Open-Angle Glaucoma Patients: Clinical Outcomes. *J. Clin. Med.* **2021**, *10*, 1628. https://doi.org/10.3390/jcm10081628

Academic Editor: Georgios Labiris

Received: 18 March 2021
Accepted: 8 April 2021
Published: 12 April 2021

Publisher's Note: MDPI stays neutral with regard to jurisdictional claims in published maps and institutional affiliations.

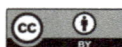

Copyright: © 2021 by the authors. Licensee MDPI, Basel, Switzerland. This article is an open access article distributed under the terms and conditions of the Creative Commons Attribution (CC BY) license (https://creativecommons.org/licenses/by/4.0/).

1. Introduction

The term glaucoma covers a wide range of multifactorial, chronic, and progressive optic neuropathies, characterized by progressive loss of retinal ganglion cells and subsequent visual field defects [1].

Glaucoma is a leading cause of irreversible blindness, and is estimated to affect over 111 million people worldwide by 2040 [2].

The main goal of glaucoma treatment is to slow the progression of the disease and to preserve, as much as possible, the patient quality of life.

Up to now, decreasing intraocular pressure (IOP) has been the only proven method to treat glaucoma [3]. To do so, different treatment strategies, such as medical therapy, laser, and surgery are currently available.

Although topical hypotensive medication is usually the first treatment approach, many patients do not achieve adequate glaucoma control due to different causes, including poor adherence, side effects, or lack of maintained efficacy [4,5].

Despite trabeculectomy being considered the gold standard in glaucoma surgery, due mainly to its well-established efficacy in terms of lowering IOP [6], it may lead to potential vision-threatening complications [7].

Minimally invasive glaucoma surgery (MIGS) devices have been developed as a safer and less traumatic means of lowering IOP in patients with glaucoma [8–11].

Among the different MIGS devices, the ab interno gel Implant XEN® (Allergan, Dublin, Ireland) allows flow of aqueous humor from the anterior chamber to the subconjunctival space [8–11].

Although many studies have shown the good efficacy/safety profile of XEN45 [12–17], the evidence assessing the outcomes of XEN63 is very limited [18–21] and those trials were done with a previous version of the device during development, which was never commercialized and differs from the current commercially available XEN63 device in many aspects (i.e., needle gauge, injector design, implantation technique, etc.).

The main difference between XEN45 and XEN63 is the bore of the stent [10,11,18–21]. The new XEN63 device is introduced by using a 27G needle, similarly to the XEN45 stent. Since the outer diameter of XEN63 is greater than that of XEN45, the side flow with the XEN63 is reduced compared with the XEN45 (Figure 1).

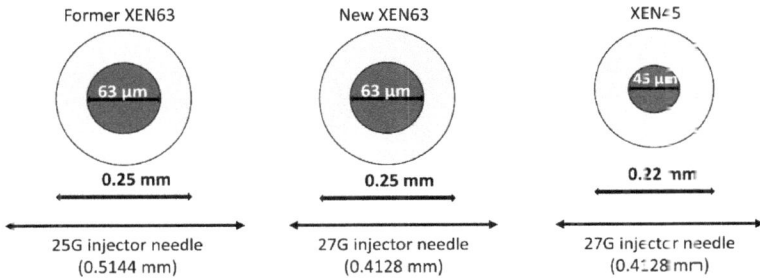

Figure 1. A comparison of the outer and inner diameters of the former XEN63, new XEN63, and XEN45 devices. The former XEN63 device was inserted by using a 25G needle injector (with an outer diameter of 0.5144 mm), while the new XEN63 device is inserted by using a 27G needle injector (with an outer diameter of 0.4128 mm, which is 19.8% smaller). As compared to XEN45 implant, the outer diameter of XEN63 is only 12% greater, while the inner diameter is 1.4 times greater. Since the new XEN63 and the XEN45 devices are inserted by using a 27G injector needle, the side flow with the XEN63 is reduced compared with the XEN45.

The new XEN63 device was developed for decreasing the incision site as compared to the former XEN63 device, and at the same time increasing the aqueous humor flow rate as compared to XEN45, which would provide lower IOPs.

The purpose of this study is to assess the efficacy in terms of IOP lowering and reduction in number of ocular hypotensive drugs of the upcoming new model of XEN63 stent implant. Additionally, the current study also aimed to evaluate the incidence of adverse events in the early postoperative period.

2. Materials and Methods

2.1. Design

Retrospective, open-label, and bicenter clinical study.

The study protocol was approved by the Ethic Committee of the University of Torino, which waived the need for written informed consent. The study was conducted in accordance with the principles of the Declaration of Helsinki.

2.2. Patients

The study was conducted on consecutive OAG patients who underwent a XEN63 implant, either alone or in combination with cataract surgery, between February and June 2020.

All participants were required to meet the following inclusion criteria: age ≥ 40 years, clinical diagnosis of OAG, and an unmet target IOP despite medical therapy. Patients with narrow-angle glaucoma (unless the surgeon believed that there was sufficient space to safely implant the device), severe conjunctival scars, ocular pemphigoid, phacodonesis, progressive retinal or optic nerve disease of any cause, or history of major ocular surgery (except phacoemulsification) within the previous 6 months were excluded from the study.

2.3. Device

In the current study, a MIGS device (Allergan, Irvine, CA, USA) was used. It is composed of porcine gelatin crosslinked with glutaraldehyde. The stent is 6 mm in length, with an outer diameter of 250 μm and an inner diameter of 63 μm.

2.4. Surgical Technique

All the surgical procedures were performed, under local anesthesia, by the same two experienced surgeons (AMF and MF).

The XEN implant was placed in the superior nasal quadrant using a standard ab interno technique [16,17,20]. After anesthesia and skin disinfection, conjunctival upper-nasal quadrant was marked 3 mm from the limbus. Before surgery, 0.1 mL of mitomycin C (MMC) 0.02–0.03% was injected intra-tenon in the supero-nasal quadrant.

After injecting a viscoelastic with high cohesivity, the pre-loaded injector needle was inserted at the inferotemporal quadrant through a 1.8 mm corneal paracentesis. An intraoperative goniolens was used to verify placement through the non-pigmented part of the trabecular meshwork. Once the goniolens was removed, the tip was advanced approximately 3 mm through the sclera, and the implant was finally positioned into the subconjunctival space. The position of the implant in the anterior chamber was checked, by gonioscopy, before removing the viscoelastic. In order to confirm the lack of adhesions, sideways movements of the implant were performed until it moved freely under the conjunctiva.

Afterwards, implant function and bleb formation were assessed by constant irrigation with balanced salt solution (BSS). Finally, the corneal incisions were hydrated with BSS.

In eyes that underwent cataract surgery, phacoemulsification was performed using the surgeon's preferred technique and XEN63 was implanted in all cases after cataract surgery.

Perioperative care included antibiotic therapy 4 times a day for 1 week and anti-inflammatory therapy with steroids 6 times daily, which was slowly tapered over three months.

At baseline, each subject underwent a standard ophthalmic exam, which included a detailed medical history, anterior segment and fundus examination, best corrected visual acuity (BCVA), IOP measurement assessed at 9 am (± 1 h) using Goldmann applanation tonometry, and gonioscopy. A computerized visual field (Humphrey visual field analyzer; Carl Zeiss Meditec, Dublin, CA, USA) performed within 6 months before XEN63 implantation was considered as the baseline examination.

Follow-up visits included anterior segment examination, paying special attention to filtering bleb, BCVA, IOP, dilated fundus examination, and the incidence of adverse events.

Topical and systemic IOP-lowering medications were suspended on the day of surgery.

Patients with bleb fibrosis, flat bleb, and/or elevated IOP underwent needling, which was performed in the theater.

Special attention was paid to avoid or delay ocular hypotensive drug reintroduction as much as possible. Before starting any postoperative antiglaucoma medications, surgeons performed either needling or bleb revision. If this approach failed or the patient refused to undergo these procedures, topical hypotensive medication was reintroduced.

2.5. Outcomes

Primary endpoints were the IOP at month 3 and the incidence of serious adverse events.

Secondary endpoints included incidence of any adverse event, reduction in number of ocular hypotensive medications from baseline to month 3, proportion of patients achieving an IOP lowering $\geq 30\%$ and $\geq 20\%$ without antiglaucoma medications, proportion of patients achieving a final IOP ≤12 mm Hg, ≤14 mm Hg, ≤16 mm Hg, or ≤18 mm Hg without medications, and incidence of non-serious adverse events.

2.5. Statistical Analysis

A standard statistical analysis was performed using Prism 9 version 9.0 (GraphPad Software; San Diego, CA, USA).

Although sample size was not calculated before the study, we conducted a post hoc analysis for testing the adequacy of the sample. The post hoc power analyses was determined for an alpha level of 0.05, the study sample size, and the effect size observed in the study [22].

Data are expressed as number (percentage), mean ± standard deviation (SD), or mean (95% confidence interval, CI) as appropriate.

Data were tested for normal distribution using a Shapiro–Wilks test.

Changes in IOP and number of ocular hypotensive medications were performed by means of repeated measures ANOVA and the Greenhouse–Geisser correction test.

The last-observation-carried-forward method was used to impute missing data.

A p value of less than 0.05 was considered significant.

3. Results

Twenty-three patients met the inclusion/exclusion criteria requirements.

Mean age was 67.8 ± 15.3 years and 15 (65.2%) were women. Table 1 shows the main baseline clinical and demographic characteristics of the study population.

Table 1. Main baseline clinical and demographic characteristics of the study sample.

Variable	Overall (n = 23)	XEN 63 (n = 20)	Phaco + XEN63 (n = 3)
Age, years			
Mean ± SD	67.8 ± 15.3	67.3 ± 15.9	71.3 ± 12.4
Sex, n (%)			
Women	15 (65.2)	14 (70.0)	1 (33.3)
Men	8 (34.8)	6 (30.0)	2 (66.7)
Type of glaucoma			
POAG	14 (60.9)	12 (60.0)	2 (66.7)
Uveitic	4 (17.4)	3 (15.0)	1 (33.3)
PXG	1 (4.3)	1 (5.0)	0 (0.0)
PACG	1 (4.3)	1 (5.0)	0 (0.0)
Traumatic	1 (4.3)	1 (5.0)	0 (0.0)
Missing information	2 (8.7)	2 (10.0)	0 (0.0)
Previous laser, n (%)			
No	21 (91.3)	18 (90.0)	3 (100.0)
SLT	1 (4.3)	1 (5.0)	0 (0.0)
Nd:YAG Iridotomy	1 (4.3)	1 (5.0)	0 (0.0)
Previous surgery *, n (%)			
None	2 (8.7)	0 (0.0)	3 (100.0)
Cataract	14 (60.9)	14 (70.0)	0 (0.0)
Refractive (laser)	3 (13.0)	3 (15.0)	0 (0.0)
Trabecular MIG	2 (8.7)	2 (10.0)	0 (0.0)
Subconjunctival MIG	2 (8.7)	2 (10.0)	0 (0.0)
BCVA, ETDRS			
Mean ± SD	0.49 ± 0.26	0.54 ± 0.24	0.23 ± 0.15
ECC			
Mean ± SD	2217.9 ± 343.1	2223.4 ± 297.0	2151.0 ± 563.8

Table 1. *Cont.*

Variable	Overall (*n* = 23)	XEN 63 (*n* = 20)	Phaco + XEN63 (*n* = 3)
MD, dB Mean ± SD	−17.03 ± 9.96	−16.71 ± 10.51	−18.23 ± 9.44
PSD, dB Mean ± SD	7.00 ± 2.28	7.10 ± 3.08	6.66 ± 3.2
NTOHM Mean ± SD	2.27 ± 0.94	2.26 ± 0.99	2.33 ± 0.58
IOP, mm Hg Mean ± SD	27.0 ± 7.8	26.5 ± 8.2	30.3 ± 3.2

* Patients may have undergone more than one procedure. Abbreviations: Phaco: Phacoemulsification; SD: Standard deviation; POAG: Primary open-angle glaucoma; PXG: Pseudoexfolitive glaucoma; PACG: Primary angle-closure glaucoma; SLT: Selective laser trabeculoplasty; YAG: Neodymium-doped Yttrium Aluminium Garnet; MIG: Minimally invasive glaucoma device; BCVA: Best corrected visual acuity; ETDRS: Early treatment diabetic retinopathy study; ECC: Endothelial cell count; MD: Mean defect; PSD: Pattern standard deviation; NTOHM: Number of topical ocular hypotensive medications; IOP: Intraocular pressure.

In the overall study population, baseline IOP was significantly reduced from 27.0 ± 7.8 mm Hg to 12.2 ± 3.4 mm Hg at month 3 ($p < 0.0001$) (Figure 2).

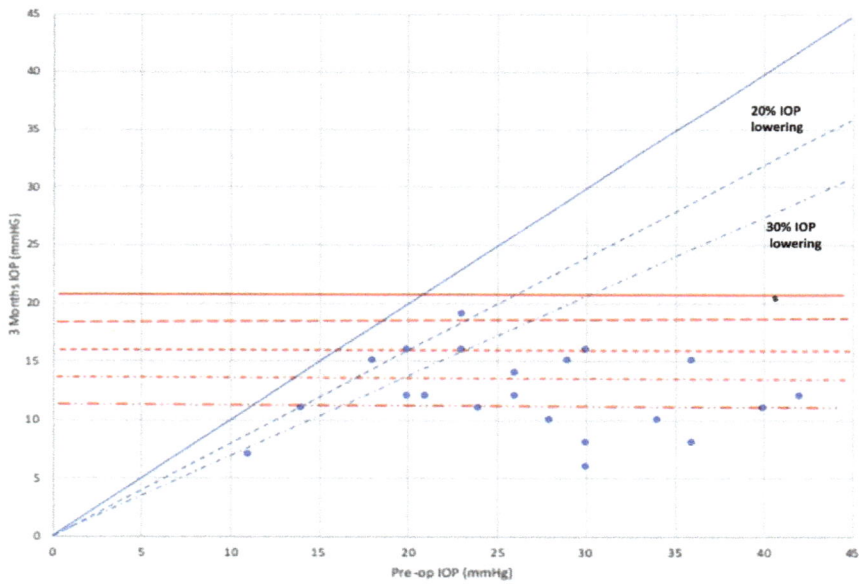

Figure 2. Scatter plot of the intraocular pressure at baseline and month 3. Mean difference −14.8 ± 6.0 mm Hg, 95 Confidence interval −18.4 to −11.2 mm Hg; $p < 0.0001$ (two-tailed paired-samples Student *t* test). The 20% and the 30% lines indicate the level beneath which an IOP reduction of more than 20% or 30%, respectively, compared to baseline value before surgery was reached by the individual cases. IOP: Intraocular pressure.

Figure 3 shows the mean IOP over the course of the study follow-up.

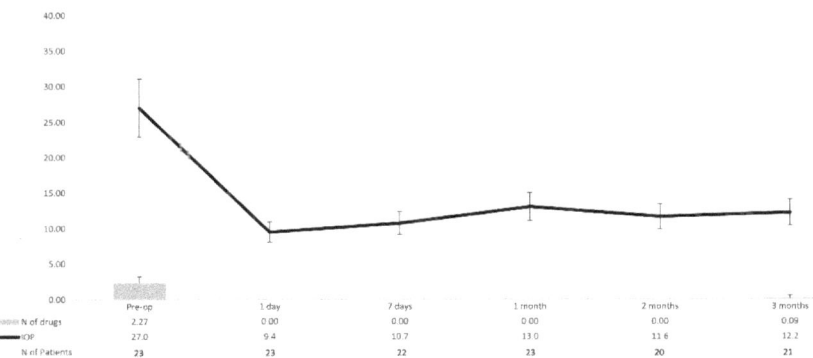

Figure 3. Overview of the mean intraocular pressure (IOP) and number of hypotensive medications over the course of the study follow-up in the overall study population. Vertical bars represent standard deviation. IOP: Intraocular pressure.

When compared to baseline, mean (95% confidence interval) IOP lowering was −17.6 (−22.0 to −13.1) mm Hg, $p < 0.0001$; −16.3 (−20.8 to −11.8) mm Hg, $p < 0.0001$; −14.0 (−18.6 to −9.4) mm Hg, $p < 0.0001$, −15.4 (−20.2 to −10.6) mm Hg, $p < 0.0001$; and −14.8 (−20.1 to −9.5) mm Hg, $p < 0.0001$ at day 1, day 7, and months 1, 2, and 3, respectively.

At month-3, mean lowering IOP was 40.8 ± 23.5%, with 14 (60.9%) and 16 (69.6%) eyes achieving an IOP lowering ≥30% and ≥20% without hypotensive medication, respectively.

Mean number of topical ocular hypotensive medications was significantly reduced from 2.27 ± 0.94 drugs at baseline to 0.09 ± 0.42 drugs at month 3 ($p < 0.0001$). At month 3, 22 (95.7%) eyes did not receive any antiglaucoma medication.

BCVA did not change over the course of the study (mean change: 0.1 ± 0.2).

At day-7, 4 (17.4%) eyes showed a ≥2-line worsening in BCVA as compared to baseline, where two of them belonged to the combo group (Table 2).

Table 2. Overview of the number (%) of patients who experienced changes in best corrected visual acuity throughout the study.

	Day 1	Day 7	Month 1	Month 3
Worse ≥2 lines, n (%)	4 (17.4)	4 (17.4)	2 (8.7)	2 (8.7)
Worse ≥1 line, n (%)	5 (26.1)	7 (30.4)	3 (13.0)	3 (13.0)
Unchanged, n (%)	9 (39.1)	6 (26.1)	8 (34.8)	6 (26.1)
Improvement ≥1 line, n (%)	0 (0.0)	2 (8.7)	3 (13.0)	2 (8.7)
Improvement ≥2 lines, n (%)	4 (17.4)	4 (17.4)	7 (30.4)	8 (34.8)

Regarding safety, four (17.4%) eyes had hypotony (an IOP ≤ 6 mm Hg) at postoperative day one, which was successfully resolved without sequelae and resolved with medical therapy within a month. Three (13.0%) eyes required needling over the course of the study follow-up (mean time for needling 35.6 ± 9.7 days), one eye with mitomycin-c and two with 5-fluorouracil. Only one eye underwent needling due to elevated IOP. Five (21.7%) eyes underwent digital ocular massage. One (4.3%) eye had anterior chamber bleeding during the surgery, one (4.3%) eye had a 1.5 mm hyphema at day 1, and 4 (17.4%) had choroidal detachment (3 at day 7 and 1 at day 15), which was successfully resolved with medical treatment, at the month-1 visit.

4. Discussion

Over the past several years there has been growing interest in MIGS devices, mainly due to the need for a safer alternative to traditional surgery.

According to the results of the collaborative initial glaucoma treatment study (CIGTS) [7], trabeculectomy was associated with a fifty percent incidence of early postoperative complications. In the same study, choroidal detachment, anterior chamber bleeding, or anterior chamber flattening had an incidence equal to or greater than 10% [7].

Additionally, the results of the tube versus trabeculectomy study showed that the rate of early postoperative complications (those developed within the first month after surgery) was 37% in the trabeculectomy group [23].

According to the results of the current study, even if they are limited to only 23 eyes and with short follow-up of 3 months, XEN63 provided a better IOP lowering effect than XEN45 [12–17,24–27].

It is important to mention the good hypotensive profile found in our study, with a mean IOP lowering of 40.8 ± 23.5% and 16 (69.6%) eyes achieving an IOP lowering ≥30% without hypotensive medication.

The XEN45 implant has shown a good early and long-term postoperative safety profile, while maintaining good IOP lowering [12–17].

When comparing our results with other studies, which reported IOP data of XEN45 stent at month-3, it can be observed that the mean IOP achieved with XEN63 was consistently lower (see Table 3). The same holds true if we examine the differential reduction in pressure [15,26] (Table 3).

Table 3. Overview of the intraocular pressure (IOP) and number of hypotensive medications in eyes that underwent XEN45 implant surgery in different studies at month-3.

Study	MMC	Type of Glaucoma	Baseline IOP, mm Hg	M3 IOP, mm Hg	IOP Lowering (%)	IOP Lowering, mm Hg	Mean Pre-operative Medications	Mean Post-operative Medications at M3	Needling Rates at the End of the Study, n (%)
Reitsamer et al. [13]	10–80 µg/mL [1]	POAG	21.4 (3.6) *	15.7 [†]	−25.0 [†]	N.A.	2.7 (0.9)	0.5 (0.9)	83 (41.1)
Marcos-Parra et al. [15]	10 µg/mL	OAG [3]	19.1 (5.4) *	N.A.	N.A.	−6.1 (−9.9 to −0.1) **	2.5 (0.8)	N.A.	13 (20.0)
Fea et al. [16]	20 µg/mL	OAG [3]	23.9 (7.6) *	15.1 [†]	N.A.	N.A.	3.0 (1.0)	0.4 [†]	79 (46.2)
Grover et al. [24]	20 µg/mL [2]	Refractory OAG [3]	25.1 (3.7) *	16.6 (5.5) *	−32.7 [†]	−8.5 [†]	3.5 (1.0)	0.5 [†]	21 (32.3)
Ibáñez-Muñoz et al. [25]	10 µg/mL	OAG [3]	22.8 (20.8 to 24.7) **	16.4 (14.3 to 18.5) **	N.A.	N.A.	3.4 (0.8)	N.A.	19 (26.0)
Laborda-Guirao et al. [26]	20 µg/mL	OAG [3]	21.0 (5.2) *	14.5 (13.6 to 15.4) **	N.A.	−6.7 (−8.8 to −4.6)	2.8 (2.7 to 3.0) **	N.A.	7 (8.8)
Theilig et al. [27]	10 µg/mL	POAG	24.5 (6.7) *	16.8 (6.3)	N.A.	N.A.	3.0 (1.1) *	1.1 (1.4) *	42 (42.0)
Hengerer et al. [28]	10 µg/mL	OAG [4]	32.2 (9.1) *	14.6 [†]	N.A.	N.A.	3.1 (1.0) *	−2.7 (1.2) [‡]	67 (27.7) ***
Current study	20–30 µg/mL [1]	OAG [3]	27.0 (7.8) *	12.2 (3.4) *	−40.8 (23.5) *	−14.8 (−20.1 to −9.5) **	2.3 (0.9) *	0.1 (0.4) *	3 (13.0)

* Mean (Standard deviation); ** Mean (95% confidence interval); [†] Data about standard deviation was not provided; [‡] Mean reduction from baseline; *** All the needling procedures were done between week 1 and month 3; Abbreviations: MMC: Mitomycin C; IOP: Intraocular pressure; M: Month; POAG: Primary open-angle glaucoma, OAG: Open-angle glaucoma; NA: Not available. [1] MMC dose at the surgeon's discretion (2 patients received 5-fluorouracil); [2] Sponges saturated with MMC; [3] It includes primary and secondary open-angle glaucoma; [4] Besides open-angle glaucoma patients, it included patients with uveitic glaucoma, angle closure glaucoma, and neovascular glaucoma.

With the exception of the Hengerer et al. study [28], the baseline IOP of our study was higher than that reported by other authors [13,15,16,24–27]. Despite its short-term follow-up, this study points to the fact that XEN 63, is not only able to achieve lower IOP but also that a greater lumen size of the device may benefit patients with a higher baseline pressure.

The relevance of this finding critically depends on whether early post-operative pressures may be predictive of long-term success. We have evidence suggesting that lower IOP in the early postoperative period was associated with successful outcomes in patients undergoing trabeculectomy [29,30]. Moreover, these findings seem to be applicable to the XEN45 device [16,31]. In a previous study conducted by our group [16], week-1 and month-1 postoperative IOP significantly correlated with the final IOP and those eyes with a lower IOP at week 1 had a higher success rate.

Currently available scientific evidence evaluating the efficacy and safety of the XEN63 implant is very limited and information about the former device was never commercially available [18–21]. Although in general terms the results of these studies have shown good efficacy and safety profile of the former device, due to differences in the surgical technique and the device, it is difficult to compare our results with those of the previous XEN63 studies.

The main difference between the former XEN63 device and the new one is the surgical technique. While the former XEN63 stent was implanted through a 2.2 mm peripheral corneal incision with a 25G injector needle, the new XEN63 device is implanted through a 1.8 mm corneal paracentesis by using a 27G injector needle (see Figure 1). This new surgical approach reduces the side flow of the new XEN63 as compared with the former one. Additionally, previous studies were performed without MMC [18–21].

Regarding safety, the most commonly reported adverse event was choroidal detachment (4 eyes), which was successfully resolved without treatment at the month-1 visit.

In this study, four (17.4%) eyes had an IOP ≤ 6 mm Hg at postoperative day one, but they were resolved without consequences.

On this subject, Lenzhofer et al. [19], using the former XEN63 device, reported that 3 (4.7%) eyes required some intervention (between surgery and end of the study) due to low IOP. Additionally, Lavin-Dapena et al. [21], also evaluating the former XEN63 device, found hypotony (similar criterion than ours) in 3 (27.3%) eyes at day 1. However, it should be noted that both studies did not use MMC, which in theory might reduce the incidence of hypotony.

This brings us to the question of whether the better IOP lowering effect obtained with XEN63 would theoretically be associated with a greater risk of hypotony.

Despite the greater inner diameter of XEN63, the incidence of hypotony was not significantly different than that observed with XEN45 [12–17]. This may be because the resistance is determined by the subconjunctival bleb [20]. Another explanation may be related to our surgical technique. Since the needle caliper used to make the track through the sclera is smaller than the previous one, the risk of peritubular filtration should not be greater than with XEN45.

Avoidance of hypotony in the early post-operative phase following glaucoma drainage device surgery is paramount if serious complications are to be avoided. Hypotony in the early postoperative period is a common and significant complication that has been associated with delayed visual recovery following trabeculectomy [32,33]. The reason why early post-operative complications are lower than in trabeculectomy may be due to the fact that the pre-determined lumen allows for a much more controlled outflow as compared to the traditional filtration surgery. Although restriction of outflow using different suturing techniques can improve the safety profile and reduce the rate of early complications observed with trabeculectomy, this carries the disadvantage of manipulation of the sutures in the post-operative period [34].

In this study, early hypotony was not related to ocular complications or visual acuity loss. In the overall study sample, mean visual acuity did not change over the course of the study. Although at day-7, 4 (17.4%) eyes had a $\geq$2-line worsening in BCVA as compared to baseline, two eyes recovered within a month.

Moreover, it should be highlighted that at month 3, eight (34.8%) eyes showed a $\geq$2-line improvement in BCVA as compared to baseline.

Unfortunately, as far as we know, visual acuity changes have not been reported in detail in previous studies, beyond its relationship with hypotonic maculopathy. This issue makes it extremely difficult to compare our results with other studies.

Vision loss associated with hypotony can be bothersome especially for one-eyed patients. Studies comparing the different kinds of glaucoma treatment using quality of life as an outcome are rare. However, patients that have undergone trabeculectomy have reported a worsening in quality of life in the early postoperative stage, which was directly linked to the local effects of the surgery [35].

Regarding needling, in the present study, 3 (13.0%) eyes underwent post-operative needling, which was a low rate compared to that reported in previous XEN45 papers [12–17]. Moreover, it should be noted that in 2 out of these 3 cases, needling was performed as a preventive measure and not because of a frank elevation of IOP.

The current study has several limitations that should be taken into consideration when assessing its results. The first one is its retrospective design. Potential bias and confounding factors are inherent of retrospective studies. Nevertheless, selection of strict inclusion/exclusion criteria tried to minimize their impact. The second limitation is its limited follow-up time. Nevertheless, the assessment of short-term clinical outcomes may be useful, since early postoperative IOP seems to be associated with the success of the procedure. The third limitation is the lack of sample size calculation before starting the study. However, according to the results of the study, the power for detecting mean IOP lowering and ocular hypotensive drug reduction, between baseline and month 3, was 99% for each. Finally, the last limitation was the lack of a control group. It would have been interesting to conduct a head-to-head comparison, preferably a randomized clinical trial, between XEN45 and XEN63.

5. Conclusions

The results of the current study clearly suggested that XEN63 was an effective and safe surgical procedure in OAG patients. XEN63 significantly lowered IOP and reduced the number of antiglaucoma medications, with a good safety profile. Its limited incidence of hypotony, in combination with a better understanding of the use of MMC (both in terms of concentration and area of injection), may allow physicians to treat more advanced patients and to obtained a lower target-IOP in the long-term.

Further research is needed to assess its long-term clinical outcomes, as well as to identify potential factors associated with clinical success.

Author Contributions: Conceptualization, methodology, funding acquisition, supervision, and review and editing the manuscript, A.M.F.; Validation, methodology, and project administration, M.M., Investigation and data curation, A.R.; Investigation and data curation, C.P.; Investigation, software, and formal analysis, L.M.; Conceptualization, methodology, funding acquisition, supervision, and review and editing the manuscript, M.F. All authors have read and agreed to the published version of the manuscript.

Funding: The authors wish to acknowledge Allergan for their support with the with the medical writing. It should be noted that Allergan was not involved in the preparation of the manuscript nor did the company influence in any way the scientific conclusions reached. Editorial assistance in the preparation of this manuscript was provided by Antonio Martinez MD (Ciencia y Deporte S.L.). Support for this assistance was funded by Allergan, an AbbVie company.

Institutional Review Board Statement: The study protocol was approved by the Ethic Committee of the University of Torino, which waived the need for written informed consent.

Informed Consent Statement: The local ethics committee waived the need for written informed consent of the participants.

Data Availability Statement: The data presented in this study are available on reasonable request from the corresponding author.

Acknowledgments: Medical writing and Editorial assistant services have been provided by Ciencia y Deporte S.L. and covered by a Grant from Allergan. Support for this assistance was funded by Allergan, an AbbVie company.

Conflicts of Interest: Dr Fea has received a Grant from Allergan during the conduct of the study. None of the Co-authors have any conflict of interest to declare.

References

1. Weinreb, R.N.; Khaw, P.T. Primary open-angle glaucoma. *Lancet* **2004**, *363*, 1711–1720. [CrossRef]
2. Tham, Y.C.; Li, X.; Wong, T.Y.; Quigley, H.A.; Aung, T.; Cheng, C.Y. Global prevalence of glaucoma and projections of glaucoma burden through 2040: A systematic review and meta-analysis. *Ophthalmology* **2014**, *121*, 2081–2090. [CrossRef]
3. Boland, M.V.; Ervin, A.M.; Friedman, D.S.; Jampel, H.D.; Hawkins, B.S.; Vollenweider, D.; Chelladurai, Y.; Ward, D.; Suarez-Cuervo, C.; Robinson, K.A. Comparative effectiveness of treatments for open-angle glaucoma: A systematic review for the U.S. Preventive Services Task Force. *Ann. Intern. Med.* **2013**, *158*, 271–279. [CrossRef]
4. Newman-Casey, P.A.; Robin, A.L.; Blachley, T.; Farris, K.; Heisler, M.; Resnicow, K.; Lee, P.P. The Most Common Barriers to Glaucoma Medication Adherence: A Cross-Sectional Survey. *Ophthalmology* **2015**, *122*, 1308–1316. [CrossRef] [PubMed]
5. Lichter, P.R.; Musch, D.C.; Gillespie, B.W.; Guire, K.E.; Janz, N.K.; Wren, P.A.; Richard, M.P.H.; CIGTS Study Group. Interim clinical outcomes in the Collaborative Initial Glaucoma Treatment Study comparing initial treatment randomized to medications or surgery. *Ophthalmology* **2001**, *108*, 1943–1953. [CrossRef]
6. Landers, J.; Martin, K.; Sarkies, N.; Bourne, R.; Watson, P. A twenty-year follow-up study of trabeculectomy: Risk factors and outcomes. *Ophthalmology* **2012**, *119*, 694–702. [CrossRef]
7. Jampel, H.D.; Musch, D.C.; Gillespie, B.W.; Lichter, P.R.; Wright, M.M.; Guire, K.E.; Collaborative Initial Glaucoma Treatment Study Group. Perioperative complications of trabeculectomy in the collaborative initial glaucoma treatment study (CIGTS). *Am. J. Ophthalmol.* **2005**, *140*, 16–22. [CrossRef] [PubMed]
8. Lavia, C.; Dallorto, L.; Maule, M.; Ceccarelli, M.; Fea, A.M. Minimally-invasive glaucoma surgeries (MIGS) for open angle glaucoma: A systematic review and meta-analysis. *PLoS ONE* **2017**, *12*, e0183142. [CrossRef] [PubMed]
9. Ansari, E. An Update on Implants for Minimally Invasive Glaucoma Surgery (MIGS). *Ophthalmol. Ther.* **2017**, *6*, 233–241. [CrossRef]
10. Pillunat, L.E.; Erb, C.; Jünemann, A.G.; Kimmich, F. Micro-invasive glaucoma surgery (MIGS): A review of surgical procedures using stents. *Clin. Ophthalmol.* **2018**, *12*, 287. [CrossRef] [PubMed]
11. Chaudhary, A.; Salinas, L.; Guidotti, J.; Mermoud, A.; Mansouri, K. XEN Gel Implant: A new surgical approach in glaucoma. *Expert Rev. Med. Devices* **2018**, *15*, 47–59. [CrossRef]
12. De Gregorio, A.; Pedrotti, E.; Russo, L.; Morselli, S. Minimally invasive combined glaucoma and cataract surgery: Clinical results of the smallest ab interno gel stent. *Int. Ophthalmol.* **2018**, *38*, 1129–1134. [CrossRef]
13. Reitsamer, H.; Sng, C.; Vera, V.; Lenzhofer, M.; Barton, K.; Stalmans, I.; Apex Study Group. Two-year results of a multicenter study of the ab interno gelatin implant in medically uncontrolled primary open-angle glaucoma. *Graefes Arch. Clin. Exp. Ophthalmol.* **2019**, *257*, 983–996. [CrossRef]
14. Chatzara, A.; Chronopoulou, I.; Theodossiadis, G.; Theodossiadis, P.; Chatziralli, I. XEN Implant for Glaucoma Treatment: A Review of the Literature. *Semin. Ophthalmol.* **2019**, *34*, 93–97. [CrossRef] [PubMed]
15. Marcos-Parra, M.T.; Salinas-López, J.A.; López-Grau, N.S.; Ceausescu, A.M.; Pérez-Santonja, J.J. XEN implant device versus trabeculectomy, either alone or in combination with phacoemulsification, in open-angle glaucoma patients. *Graefes Arch. Clin. Exp. Ophthalmol.* **2019**, *257*, 1741–1750. [CrossRef] [PubMed]
16. Fea, A.M.; Bron, A.M.; Economou, M.A.; Laffi, G.; Martini, E.; Figus, M.; Oddone, F. European study of the efficacy of a cross-linked gel stent for the treatment of glaucoma. *J. Cataract Refract. Surg.* **2020**, *46*, 441–450. [CrossRef] [PubMed]
17. Fea, A.M.; Durr, G.M.; Marolo, P.; Malinverni, L.; Economou, M.A.; Ahmed, I. XEN® Gel Stent: A Comprehensive Review on Its Use as a Treatment Option for Refractory Glaucoma. *Clin. Ophthalmol.* **2020**, *14*, 1805–1832. [CrossRef] [PubMed]
18. Sheybani, A.; Lenzhofer, M.; Hohensinn, M.; Reitsamer, H.; Ahmed, I.I. Phacoemulsification combined with a new ab interno gel stent to treat open-angle glaucoma: Pilot study. *J. Cataract Refract. Surg.* **2015**, *41*, 1905–1909. [CrossRef] [PubMed]
19. Lenzhofer, M.; Kersten-Gomez, I.; Sheybani, A.; Gulamhusein, H.; Strohmaier, C.; Hohensinn, M.; Dick, H.B.; Hitzl, W.; Eisenkopf, L.; Sedarous, F.; et al. Four-year results of a minimally invasive transscleral glaucoma gel stent implantation in a prospective multi-centre study. *Clin. Exp. Ophthalmol.* **2019**, *47*, 581–587. [CrossRef] [PubMed]
20. Fernández-García, A.; Zhou, Y.; García-Alonso, M.; Andrango, H.D.; Poyales, F.; Garzón, N. Comparing Medium-Term Clinical Outcomes following XEN® 45 and XEN® 63 Device Implantation. *J. Ophthalmol.* **2020**, *2020*, 4796548. [CrossRef]
21. Lavin-Dapena, C.; Cordero-Ros, R.; D'Anna, O.; Mogollón, I. XEN 63 gel stent device in glaucoma surgery: A 3-years follow-up prospective study. *Eur. J. Ophthalmol.* **2020**, 1120672120952033. [CrossRef]
22. Yuan, K.-H.; Maxwell, S. On the Post Hoc Power in Testing Mean Differences. *J. Educ. Behav. Stat.* **2005**, *30*, 141–167. [CrossRef]
23. Gedde, S.J.; Herndon, L.W.; Brandt, J.D.; Budenz, D.L.; Feuer, W.J.; Schiffman, J.C.; Tube Versus Trabeculectomy Study Group. Postoperative complications in the Tube Versus Trabeculectomy (TVT) study during five years of follow-up. *Am. J. Ophthalmol.* **2012**, *153*, 804–814.e1. [CrossRef]
24. Grover, D.S.; Flynn, W.J.; Bashford, K.P.; Lewis, R.A.; Duh, Y.J.; Nangia, R.S.; Niksch, B. Performance and Safety of a New Ab Interno Gelatin Stent in Refractory Glaucoma at 12 Months. *Am. J. Ophthalmol.* **2017**, *183*, 25–36. [CrossRef] [PubMed]
25. Ibáñez-Muñoz, A.; Soto-Biforcos, V.S.; Chacón-González, M.; Rúa-Galisteo, O.; Santos, A.A.-L.; Lizuain-Abadía, M.E.; Mayor, J.L.D.R. One-year follow-up of the XEN® implant with mitomycin-C in pseudoexfoliative glaucoma patients. *Eur. J. Ophthalmol.* **2019**, *29*, 309–314. [CrossRef]
26. Laborda-Guirao, T.; Cubero-Parra, J.M.; Hidalgo-Torres, A. Efficacy and safety of XEN 45 gel stent alone or in combination with phacoemulsification in advanced open angle glaucoma patients: 1-year retrospective study. *Int. J. Ophthalmol.* **2020**, *13*, 1250–1256. [CrossRef] [PubMed]

27. Theilig, T.; Rehak, M.; Busch, C.; Bormann, C.; Schargus, M.; Unterlauft, J.D. Comparing the efficacy of trabeculectomy and XEN gel microstent implantation for the treatment of primary open-angle glaucoma: A retrospective monocentric comparative cohort study. *Sci. Rep.* **2020**, *10*, 19337. [CrossRef] [PubMed]
28. Hengerer, F.H.; Kohnen, T.; Mueller, M.; Conrad-Hengerer, I. Ab Interno Gel Implant for the Treatment of Glaucoma Patients With or Without Prior Glaucoma Surgery: 1-Year Results. *J. Glaucoma* **2017**, *26*, 1130–1136. [CrossRef] [PubMed]
29. Okimoto, S.; Kiuchi, Y.; Akita, T.; Tanaka, J. Using the early postoperative intraocular pressure to predict pressure control after a trabeculectomy. *J. Glaucoma* **2014**, *23*, 410–414. [CrossRef] [PubMed]
30. Esfandiari, H.; Pakravan, M.; Loewen, N.A.; Yaseri, M. Predictive value of early postoperative IOP and bleb morphology in Mitomycin-C augmented trabeculectomy. *F1000Research* **2017**, *6*, 1898. [CrossRef]
31. Karimi, A.; Lindfield, D. Is a Day 1 postoperative review following ab interno Xen gel stent surgery for glaucoma needed? *Clin. Ophthalmol.* **2018**, *12*, 2331–2335. [CrossRef] [PubMed]
32. Popovic, V. Early hypotony after trabeculectomy. *Acta Ophthalmol. Scand.* **1995**, *73*, 255–260. [CrossRef] [PubMed]
33. Saeedi, O.J.; Jefferys, J.L.; Solus, J.F.; Jampel, H.D.; Quigley, H.A. Risk factors for adverse consequences of low intraocular pressure after trabeculectomy. *J. Glaucoma* **2014**, *23*, e60–e68. [CrossRef] [PubMed]
34. Lin, S. Building a safer trabeculectomy. *Br. J. Ophthalmol.* **2006**, *90*, 4–5. [CrossRef] [PubMed]
35. Burr, J.; Azuara-Blanco, A.; Avenell, A.; Tuulonen, A. Medical versus surgical interventions for open angle glaucoma. *Cochrane Database Syst. Rev.* **2012**, *9*, CD004399. [CrossRef] [PubMed]

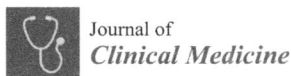

Article

Effects of Miosis on Anterior Chamber Structure in Glaucoma Implant Surgery

Kee Sup Park [1,2], Kyoung Nam Kim [1,2,*], Jaeyoung Kim [1,2], Yeon Hee Lee [1,2], Sung Bok Lee [1,2] and Chang-sik Kim [1,2]

[1] Department of Ophthalmology, Chungnam National University College of Medicine, Daejeon 35015, Korea; red-mirr@hanmail.net (K.S.P.); scullism@gmail.com (J.K.); opticalyh@hanmail.net (Y.H.L.); solee@cnu.ac.kr (S.B.L.); kcs61@cnu.ac.kr (C.-s.K.)
[2] Department of Ophthalmology, Chungnam National University Hospital, Daejeon 35015, Korea
* Correspondence: kknace@cnuh.co.kr; Tel.: +82-42-280-7604; Fax: +82-42-255-3745

Abstract: We investigated changes in anterior chamber (AC) structure after miosis in phakic eyes and pseudophakic eyes with glaucoma. In this prospective study, patients scheduled for glaucoma implant surgery were examined using anterior segment optical coherence tomography before and after miosis. Four AC parameters (AC angle, peripheral anterior chamber (PAC) depth, central anterior chamber (CAC) depth, and AC area) were analyzed before and after miosis, and then compared between phakic and pseudophakic eyes. Twenty-nine phakic eyes and 36 pseudophakic eyes were enrolled. The AC angle widened after miosis in both the phakia and pseudophakia groups ($p = 0.019$ and $p < 0.001$, respectively). In the phakia group, CAC depth ($p < 0.001$) and AC area ($p = 0.02$) were significantly reduced after miosis, and the reductions in PAC depth, CAC depth, and AC area were significantly greater than in the pseudophakia group (all $p < 0.05$). Twenty-five patients (86.2%) in the phakia group and 17 (47.2%) in the pseudophakia group had reduced CAC depth ($p = 0.004$). Although miosis increased the AC angle in both groups, AC depth decreased in most phakic eyes and a substantial number of pseudophakic eyes. Preoperative miosis before glaucoma implant surgery may interfere with implant tube placement distant from the cornea during insertion into the AC.

Keywords: pilocarpine; miosis; glaucoma implant surgery; anterior chamber

1. Introduction

The instillation of pilocarpine for the purpose of miosis may be performed before various ophthalmic surgeries or laser treatments. For example, miosis is helpful to thinly stretch the peripheral iris during peripheral laser iridotomy, prevent excessive iris resection during trabeculectomy, and prevent damage to the lens due to anterior chamber (AC) puncture and tube insertion during glaucoma implant surgery [1–4].

Glaucoma implant surgery is a common glaucoma treatment procedure. The reported surgical success rates and risks of complications are comparable with those of trabeculectomy, which is the most frequent procedure [5–7]. Although the surgical results of glaucoma implant surgery are comparable with those of trabeculectomy, concerns remain about progressive corneal endothelial damage, subsequent corneal decompensation, and resultant vision loss [3,4,8,9]. Recently, several studies using anterior segment optical coherence tomography (AS-OCT) have reported the effects on the corneal endothelium of tube insertion in the AC during glaucoma implant surgery. Koo et al. [10] and Tan et al. [11] concluded that tubes positioned closer to the cornea led to increased damage to adjacent corneal endothelium. Lee et al. reported that the angle between the tube and the cornea was narrower in eyes with significant corneal endothelial damage than in eyes without damage ($28.67 \pm 7.79°$ vs. $36.35 \pm 5.35°$, $p < 0.001$), and the distance between the tube and the cornea was shorter in eyes with corneal endothelial damage than in eyes without damage (0.98 ± 0.38 mm vs. 1.26 ± 0.39 mm, $p = 0.002$) [12]. They suggested that during its

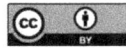

insertion into the AC, a considerable distance is required between the tube and the cornea to reduce corneal endothelial damage after glaucoma implant surgery [10–12].

In phakic eyes, pilocarpine-induced miosis reduces the AC depth in association with a reduction in AC volume and in the radius of lens curvature [13,14]. Conversely, the effects of pilocarpine in pseudophakic eyes are unclear; previous studies have yielded conflicting results [15–19]. Lea et al. [18] reported a forward shift of a rigid intraocular lens (IOL, a maximum of 0.25 mm), but found no significant change in a flexible IOL as measured by optical pachymetry. In contrast, Findl et al. [19] observed either no significant shift or a slight backward shift when using conventional three-piece IOLs, as measured by partial coherence interferometry.

Determination of the effects of preoperative miosis on AC structure, depending on the presence of phakia or pseudophakia, will help clarify whether miosis is helpful in tube placement during glaucoma implant surgery. To the best of our knowledge, no study has directly compared changes in the AC after the instillation of pilocarpine in phakic and pseudophakic eyes. Therefore, we compared changes in AC structure between phakic and pseudophakic eyes using AS-OCT after pilocarpine-induced miosis in patients scheduled for glaucoma implant surgery. Additionally, to evaluate the AC structure in relation to tube insertion, we measured the peripheral and center AC depths based on the iris surface, unlike previous studies that measured only central anterior chamber (CAC) depth based on the lens surface.

2. Methods

2.1. Patients

This prospective study was approved by the Institutional Review Board of Chungnam National University Hospital in the Republic of Korea (IRB number: 2018-03-040). It was conducted in accordance with all relevant requirements of the Declaration of Helsinki. Informed consent was acquired from all participants. Patients who were scheduled for Ahmed glaucoma valve implantation in our glaucoma clinic between June 2018 and January 2020 were consecutively enrolled in the study. Neovascular glaucoma, secondary glaucoma resulting from uveitis, ocular surgery, and glaucoma with a wide conjunctival scar from previous ocular surgery such as trabeculectomy were included as indications for Ahmed glaucoma valve implantation.

Patients were excluded if they had considerable corneal opacity that interfered with AS-OCT imaging, a fixed pupil due to iris sphincter injury or posterior synechiae, a history of acute angle closure attack, and/or evidence of zonular weakness (e.g., phacodonesis, pseudophacodonesis, and vitreous strands in the AC). Patients were also excluded if they had undergone intraocular surgery within the preceding 3 months. In each patient, the eye that met the inclusion criteria was selected. When both eyes met the criteria, one eye was selected for analysis using the random sampling method in Microsoft Excel® (Microsoft Corp., Redmond, WA, USA).

All enrolled patients underwent complete ophthalmic examinations, including best-corrected visual acuity, auto-refractometry, slit-lamp biomicroscopy, Goldmann applanation tonometry, gonioscopy, dilated fundus examination, and pachymetry (Ocuscan RxP; Alcon, Fort Worth, TX, USA), as well as measurements of axial length, AC depth, and keratometry (IOLMaster, Carl Zeiss, Jena, Germany).

2.2. Anterior Segment Optical Coherence Tomography (AS-OCT)

AS-OCT was performed before and after miosis. All patients underwent AS-OCT (Cirrus HD OCT; Carl Zeiss Meditec, Dublin, CA, USA) at the last outpatient clinic visit before glaucoma surgery. AS-OCT was performed without miosis. Subsequently, 2% pilocarpine (Alcon) was instilled twice at 5-min intervals to induce miosis. AS-OCT was repeated 50 min later. During these examinations, the patients were asked to fixate on an internal target. Images without artifacts due to eye motion and blinking were used for analysis. The scanning axis was aligned with the horizontal line passing through the center of the pupil.

Four AC parameters were acquired by AS-OCT (Figure 1). The first three parameters were measured using an integrated ruler and angle indicator: (1) AC angle (°) was defined as the angle between the corneal endothelium and anterior surface of the iris, 1 mm from the vertex of AC recess; (2) CAC depth (mm) was measured as the deepest vertical distance to the corneal endothelium following the construction of a line parallel to the horizontal line connecting the nasal to temporal scleral spur and in contact with the anterior surface of the temporal iris; and (3) peripheral anterior chamber depth (PAC depth, mm) was defined as the vertical distance from the iris surface, 2 mm from the vertex of AC recess to the corneal endothelium. Both AC angle and PAC depth were acquired from the temporal side. The fourth parameter, AC area (mm^2), was measured automatically with built-in software.

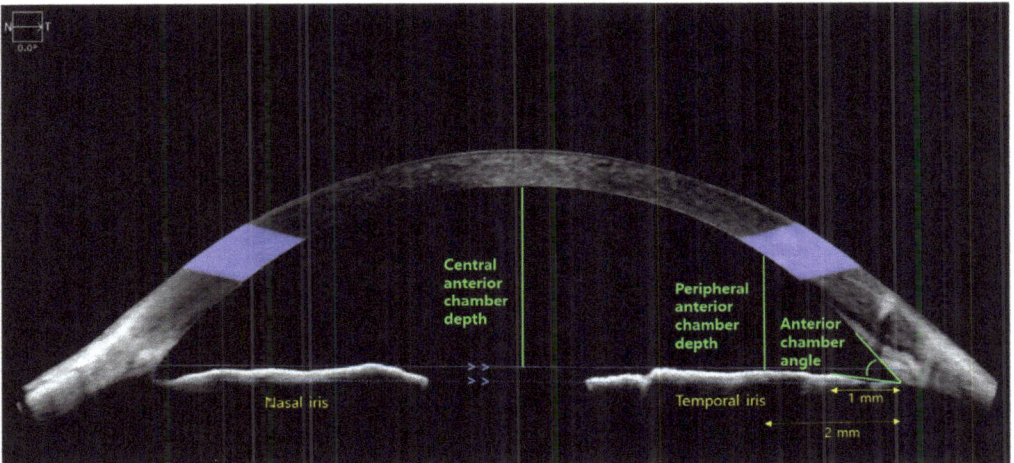

Figure 1. Anterior segment optical coherence tomography (AS-OCT) parameters. Among the four anterior chamber (AC) parameters used in this study, central anterior chamber (CAC) depth, peripheral anterior chamber (PAC) depth, and AC angle were measured using an integrated ruler and angle indicator. For the AC area, the value was measured automatically by AS-OCT.

2.3. Statistical Analysis

PASW software, version 18.0 (SPSS Inc., Chicago, IL, USA) was used for all statistical analyses. Enrolled patients were divided into two groups depending on their lens status (phakic or pseudophakic). Demographic characteristics were compared between the two groups using Student's *t*-test and Fisher's exact test. Student's *t*-test was used to compare AC parameters between the two groups. Paired *t*-tests were used to analyze post-miosis changes in AC parameters in each group, and correlations between AC parameters before and after miosis were analyzed. Differences in subgroup composition according to changes in AC parameters between two groups were analyzed using the Pearson chi-squared test. In all analyses, $p < 0.05$ was considered to indicate statistical significance.

3. Results

Data from 65 eyes of 65 patients scheduled for glaucoma implant surgery were analyzed. These included 29 phakic eyes and 36 pseudophakic eyes. The mean ages of patients in the phakia and pseudophakia groups were 62.1 ± 12.9 years and 64.8 ± 13.9 years, respectively ($p = 0.419$). The mean AC depth measured by IOLMaster, from the corneal endothelium to the anterior surface of the lens, was shallower in the phakia group than in the pseudophakia group (3.0 ± 0.6 mm vs. 4.3 ± 0.7 mm, $p < 0.001$). The mean axial lengths did not differ significantly between groups (23.4 ± 1.4 mm vs. 23.8 ± 1.2 mm, $p = 0.180$, Table 1).

Table 1. Demographic characteristics of patients.

	Phakia Group ($n = 29$)	Pseudophakia Group ($n = 36$)	p-Value *
Age (years)	62.1 ± 12.9	64.8 ± 13.9	0.419
Sex (male/female)	13/16	20/16	0.459 †
Diabetes mellitus (n)	8 (27.6%)	17 (47.2%)	0.129 †
Hypertension (n)	10 (34.5%)	16 (44.4%)	0.455 †
Type of glaucoma (n)			
Primary open-angle	11	14	
Primary angle-closure	7	5	
Uveitic	3	4	
Neovascular	5	9	
Pseudoexfoliation	3	4	
Axial length (mm)	23.4 ± 1.4	23.8 ± 1.2	0.180
Anterior chamber depth (mm)	3.0 ± 0.6	4.3 ± 0.7	<0.001
Keratometry (diopter)	44.7 ± 1.8	44.1 ± 1.5	0.131
Central corneal thickness (um)	536.5 ± 30.1	538.8 ± 24.3	0.729
Spherical equivalent (diopter)	−0.6 ± 3.6	−0.9 ± 1.2	0.695

Data are shown as mean ± standard deviation or n, * Student's t-test, † Fisher's exact test.

Table 2 compares AC parameters measured by AS-OCT between the phakia and pseudophakia groups. All AC parameters before and after miosis were significantly smaller in the phakia group (all $p < 0.001$). In the phakia group, the AC angle was wider after miosis than before miosis ($\triangle 1.48 \pm 3.21°$, $p = 0.019$). Post-miotic CAC depth ($\triangle -0.12 \pm 0.11$ mm, $p < 0.001$) and AC area ($\triangle -0.88 \pm 1.38$ mm^2, $p = 0.02$) were significantly lower than their corresponding pre-miotic values. In the pseudophakia group, AC angle was the only parameter that significantly increased after miosis ($\triangle 1.64 \pm 2.39°$, $p < 0.001$). Differences between pre- and post-miosis PAC depth, CAC depth, and AC area values were larger in the phakia group than in the pseudophakia group ($p = 0.043$, $p < 0.001$, and $p = 0.036$, respectively).

Table 2. Comparisons of anterior chamber parameters between phakia and pseudophakia groups before and after miosis.

	Phakia Group ($n = 29$)	Pseudophakia Group ($n = 36$)	p-Value *
Pre-miosis			
Anterior chamber angle (°)	28.4 ± 9.3	39.7 ± 4.0	<0.001
Peripheral anterior chamber depth (mm)	1.31 ± 0.40	1.76 ± 0.17	<0.001
Central anterior chamber depth (mm)	2.20 ± 0.62	2.86 ± 0.25	<0.001
Anterior chamber area (mm^2)	17.63 ± 5.87	23.97 ± 2.83	<0.001
Post-miosis			
Anterior chamber angle (°)	29.90 ± 7.77	41.33 ± 4.46	<0.001
Peripheral anterior chamber depth (mm)	1.26 ± 0.34	1.77 ± 0.19	<0.001
Central anterior chamber depth (mm)	2.07 ± 0.60	2.86 ± 0.27	<0.001
Anterior chamber area (mm^2)	16.76 ± 5.36	23.78 ± 3.24	<0.001
Differences †			
Anterior chamber angle (°)	1.48 ± 3.21 (0.019)	1.64 ± 2.39 (<0.001)	0.823
Peripheral anterior chamber depth (mm)	−0.06 ± 0.13 (0.571)	−0.003 ± 0.089 (0.590)	0.043
Central anterior chamber depth (mm)	−0.12 ± 0.11 (<0.001)	−0.004 ± 0.095 (0.784)	<0.001
Anterior chamber area (mm^2)	−0.88 ± 1.38 (0.02)	−0.19 ± 1.19 (0.335)	0.036

Data are shown as mean ± standard deviation, * Paired t-test, † Values indicate post-miosis−pre-miosis.

Figures 2 and 3 present the relationships between pre-miosis and post-miosis AC parameters in the phakia and pseudophakia groups, respectively. In both groups, strong positive correlations were observed in all four parameters between pre-miosis and post-miosis values (all $p < 0.001$). Correlation coefficients of the AC angle, PAC depth, and CAC depth were lower in the pseudophakia group than in the phakia group (Fisher's Z transformation, $z = 2.076$, $z = 2.535$, and $z = 2.627$; $p = 0.038$, $p = 0.011$, and $p = 0.009$, respectively). The correlation coefficient of the AC area showed a trend, but the result was not statistically significant ($z = 1.874$, $p = 0.061$).

Table 3 lists the distribution of patients stratified according to changes in AC parameters after miosis. In both groups, most patients had an enhancement of AC angle ($p = 0.678$). Most patients in the phakia group had reductions in PAC depth, CAC depth, and AC area, whereas approximately equal numbers of patients in the pseudophakia group had reductions and enhancements of those parameters ($p = 0.019$, $p = 0.002$, and $p = 0.019$, respectively).

Table 4 lists the distribution of the patients stratified according to the combination of changes in AC angle and CAC depth. In the phakia group, 19 patients (65.5%) had an enhanced AC angle and a reduced CAC depth. Six patients (20.7%) had a reduced AC angle and a reduced CAC depth. Figure 4 shows representative patients from these two subgroups (A and B, respectively). In the pseudophakia group, 19 patients (52.8%) had an enhanced AC angle and an enhanced CAC depth, and 11 patients (30.6%) had an enhanced AC angle and a reduced CAC depth ($p = 0.004$).

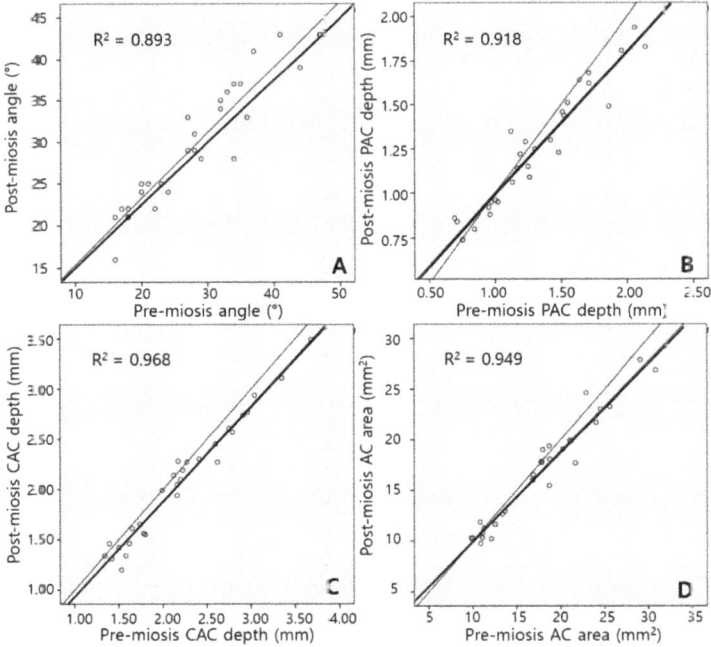

Figure 2. Scatter plots of anterior chamber (AC) parameters in the phakia group. (**A**) AC angle, (**B**) peripheral anterior chamber (PAC) depth, (**C**) central anterior chamber (CAC) depth, and (**D**) AC area. Correlations between pre-miosis and post-miosis values in all parameters were strongly positive and statistically significant (all $p < 0.001$). The thin line represents Y = X.

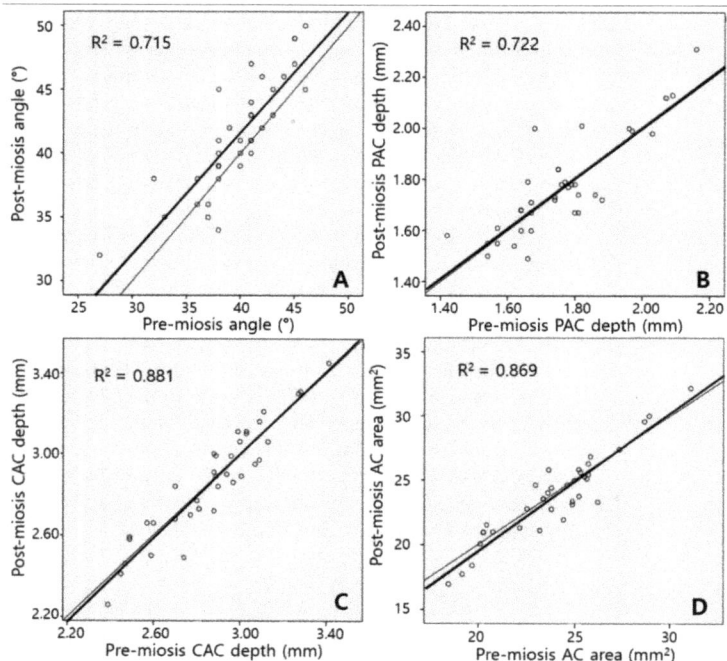

Figure 3. Scatter plots of anterior chamber (AC) parameters in the pseudophakia group. (**A**) AC angle, (**B**) peripheral anterior chamber (PAC) depth, (**C**) central anterior chamber (CAC) depth, and (**D**) AC area. Correlations between pre-miosis and post-miosis values in all parameters were positive and statistically significant (all $p < 0.001$). The thin line represents Y = X.

Table 3. Distribution of patients stratified according to changes in anterior chamber structure after miosis.

	Enhancement	Reduction	p-Value
Anterior chamber angle			
Phakia group (n)	23	6	
Pseudophakia group (n)	30	6	0.678
Peripheral anterior chamber depth			
Phakia group (n)	7	22	
Pseudophakia group (n)	19	17	0.019
Central anterior chamber depth			
Phakia group (n)	4	25	
Pseudophakia group (n)	19	17	0.002
Anterior chamber area			
Phakia group (n)	7	22	
Pseudophakia group (n)	19	17	0.019

Pearson chi-squared test.

Table 4. Distribution of patients stratified according to the combination of changes in anterior chamber angle and central anterior chamber depth after miosis.

		Phakia Group (n = 29)		Pseudophakia Group (n = 36)	
		Anterior Chamber Angle		Anterior Chamber Angle	
		Enhancement	Reduction	Enhancement	Reduction
Central anterior chamber depth	Enhancement	4 (13.8%)	0	19 (52.8%)	0
	Reduction	19 (65.5%)	6 (20.7%)	11 (30.6%)	6 (16.6%)
p-value			0.004		

Pearson chi-squared test.

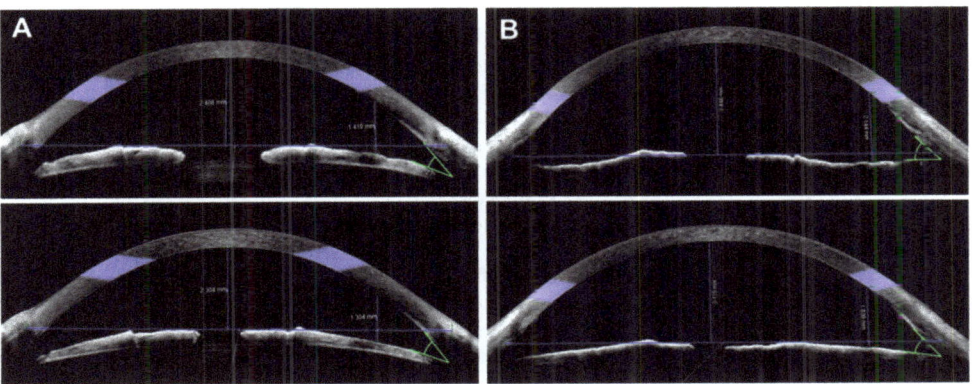

Figure 4. Anterior segment optical coherence tomography (AS-OCT) images of representative patients in the phakia group. Top depicts pre-miotic image and bottom depicts post-miotic image (**A**) Anterior chamber (AC) angle widened (27° to 32°), but central (CAC) and peripheral anterior chamber (PAC) depths became shallower after miosis (2.408 mm to 2.304 mm and 1.419 mm to 1.304 mm, respectively). (**B**) AC angle (43° to 36°) narrowed and CAC and PAC depths (3.448 to 3.115 mm and 2.144 to 1.839 mm, respectively) became shallower after miosis.

4. Discussion

We found that post-miosis changes in AC structure differed between phakic and pseudophakic eyes. In phakic eyes, most (86.2%) had a shallower AC depth after miosis, regardless of the change in AC angle. In pseudophakic eyes, the change in AC structure was relatively inconsistent. In 52.8% of patients, the AC depth became deeper and the AC angle became wider, and in 47.2% of patients, the AC depth became shallower regardless of the change in AC angle. Therefore, in considerable numbers of patients with phakia or pseudophakia, the use of pilocarpine prior to glaucoma implant surgery could adversely affect implant tube placement distant from the cornea during insertion into the AC.

Glaucoma implant surgery is increasingly being performed as an alternative or equivalent choice to trabeculectomy [5,7,20]. However, some complications such as hypotony, shallow AC, hyphema, tube–corneal contact, choroidal effusion, cataract formation, endophthalmitis, and corneal endothelial damage may result from glaucoma implant surgery [9]. Of these, progressive corneal endothelial cell loss is a major long-term complication, which leads to corneal decompensation [6,10,21]. The mechanism of corneal endothelial cell damage after glaucoma implant surgery has not been fully elucidated, but several hypotheses have been suggested. One of the most promising hypotheses is that tube insertion in the AC will affect corneal endothelial damage [9]. Some studies have yielded results to support this hypothesis. Kim et al. [22] reported that the corneal endothelial cell densities were reduced by 22.4%, 28.7%, 19.4%, and 18.3% at superior, supratemporal, supranasal, and central locations after glaucoma implant surgery. Similarly, Lee et al. [23] reported corneal endothelial cell losses of 20.3%, 22.6%, 18.1%, and 15.4% at superior, supratemporal, supranasal, and central locations, respectively. In both studies, the greatest cell loss was evident in the supratemporal location, where the tube was located. In studies using AS imaging [10–12], a shorter distance and a narrower angle between the tube and corneal endothelium were both risk factors for corneal endothelial cell loss. These results suggest that it is preferable to place the tube distant from the cornea during insertion in the AC, thereby reducing corneal endothelial damage after glaucoma implant surgery. Park et al. [24] reported that the tube in the AC gradually moved toward the corneal endothelium after glaucoma implant surgery. Therefore, it is also important to position the tube in the posterior portion of the AC to prevent long-term corneal damage after glaucoma implant surgery.

Some surgical techniques have been introduced to reduce corneal endothelial damage. Pars plana tube insertion has been performed in combination with penetrating keratoplasty when traditional AC tube insertion is not possible. However, pars plana tube insertion is only feasible in vitrectomized eyes [25–27]. Although ciliary sulcus tube insertion does not require vitrectomy, it can be used in pseudophakic eyes to avoid lens damage [28,29]. In general, during glaucoma implant surgery, the tube is inserted into the AC distant from the corneal endothelium and parallel to the front surface of the iris. Approved indications for the ophthalmic use of pilocarpine include a reduction in elevated intraocular pressure in patients with glaucoma or ocular hypertension, the prevention of postoperative elevated intraocular pressure, and the induction of miosis [30]. No consensus has been reached in terms of whether pilocarpine should be used before glaucoma implant surgery. Therefore, miosis is selectively performed in accordance with the operator's preferences. Preoperative miosis is expected to help prevent damage to the lens during AC puncture or tube insertion during surgery. However, we found that in phakic eyes, shallower AC depth is likely to hinder the insertion of the tube distant from the cornea. During tube insertion, to prevent iris incarceration into the tube opening, the tube must be inserted in parallel without contacting the iris. If the tube is inserted in a shallow AC, it will be inserted nearer to the cornea.

The administration of pilocarpine causes iris sphincter contraction, along with the contraction of the ciliary muscle, which leads to zonule relaxation and changes in both lens shape and thickness. This series of changes moves the lens-iris diaphragm forward. Therefore, the AC depth is slightly reduced [15–17]. In our study, the correlation coefficients of pre-miosis and post-miosis AC parameters were lower in pseudophakic eyes than in phakic eyes, presumably because the lens-iris diaphragm is less affected by ciliary muscle contraction in pseudophakic eyes [19]. Previous studies have demonstrated differences in post-miosis AC depth changes in pseudophakic eyes, depending on the IOL shape and material [17–19].

Rękas et al. [31] studied changes in AC configuration after cataract surgery and classified subjects into four groups based on preoperative parameters, such as the AC depth, AC angle, lens thickness, and axial length. The AC configuration was significantly different among the groups. Although these preoperative parameters are related to the amount of change in the AC after cataract surgery [32–34], Rękas et al. showed that the changes in AC depth and angle after cataract surgery explained only 42.65% of the change predicted by the preoperative parameters. Altan et al. [35] and Huang et al. [36] suggested a possible influence of other anatomical structures and postoperative changes in the eye, such as ciliary processes, ciliary zonule, and the iris. In our study, it was expected that various anatomical factors would affect the AC after miosis induced by pilocarpine instillation. However, in clinical practice, the most useful way to determine whether miosis is advantageous when preparing for glaucoma implant surgery is to directly compare the AC before and after miosis.

Considering the potential for bias, we excluded patients with zonular weakness, which is known to cause considerable change in AC depth due to miosis or mydriasis [23–25]. Importantly, patients with zonular weakness who are scheduled for surgery may have a larger reduction in AC depth than the values confirmed in this study.

This study had some limitations. First, we could not analyze whether changes in AC structure after miosis differed among subgroups according to glaucoma type because relatively few patients were enrolled. To test this hypothesis, additional studies are needed with larger numbers of patients. Second, we could not compare actual tube positions between insertion performed with and without miosis because we did not perform miosis during glaucoma implant surgery in patients if the AC angle became narrow and/or the AC depth became shallow after miosis.

In conclusion, when miosis is performed during preparation for glaucoma implant surgery, patients with phakic eyes may have a shallow AC depth that causes difficulty in positioning the tube distant from the cornea. In some patients with a considerable reduction in AC depth after miosis, cataract surgery may be considered to avoid tube insertion near the cornea. Additionally, in many pseudophakic eyes, the AC may become shallow after miosis. Therefore, if miosis is performed routinely before glaucoma implant surgery, the suitability of miosis in each patient should be checked before surgery by examining changes in the AC due to miosis.

Author Contributions: Conceptualization, K.S.P. and K.N.K.; methodology, K.N.K. and J.K.; validation, J.K., K.N.K. and Y.H.L.; formal analysis, Y.H.L., S.B.L., K.N.K. and C.-s.K.; investigation, J.K. and K.N.K.; data curation, K.S.P., S.B.L. and Y.H.L.; writing—original draft preparation, K.S.P., K.N.K., S.B.L.; writing—review and editing, J.K. and K.N.K.; supervision, K.N.K.; project administration, K.N.K.; All authors have read and agreed to the published version of the manuscript

Funding: This research was supported by the National Research Foundation of Korea (NRF). (2018R1C1B503613513).

Institutional Review Board Statement: The study was conducted according to the guidelines of the Declaration of Helsinki, and approved by the Institutional Review Board of Chungnam National University Hospital in the Republic of Korea (IRB number: 2018-03-040).

Informed Consent Statement: Informed consent was obtained from all subjects involved in the study.

Data Availability Statement: The data presented in this study are available on request from the corresponding author. The data are not publicly available due to privacy and ethical reasons.

Conflicts of Interest: The authors declare no conflict of interest.

References

1. Grierson, I.; Lee, W.R.; Abraham, S. Effects of pilocarpine on the morphology of the human outflow apparatus. *Br. J. Ophthalmol.* **1978**, *62*, 302–313.
2. Watson, P.; Barnett, F. Effectiveness of trabeculectomy in glaucoma. *Am. J. Ophthalmol.* **1975**, *79*, 831–845.
3. Shaarawy, T. *Glaucoma, Volume 2: Surgical Management*; Saunders Ltd.: Wynnewood, PA, USA, 2009.
4. Kim, J.; Lee, J.; Kee, C. Tissue incarceration after Ahmed valve implantation. *J. Korean Ophthalmol. Soc.* **2012**, *53*, 1053–1056.
5. Gedde, S.J.; Schiffman, J.C.; Feuer, W.J.; Herndon, L.W.; Brandt, J.D.; Budenz, D.L.; Group, T.v.T.S. Treatment outcomes in the Tube Versus Trabeculectomy (TVT) study after five years of follow-up. *Am. J. Ophthalmol.* **2012**, *153*, 789–803.e2.
6. Minckler, D.S.; Francis, B.A.; Hodapp, E.A.; Jampel, H.D.; Lin, S.C.; Samples, J.R.; Smith, S.D.; Singh, K. Aqueous shunts in glaucoma: A report by the American Academy of Ophthalmology. *Ophthalmology* **2008**, *115*, 1089–1098.
7. Arora, K.S.; Robin, A.L.; Corcoran, K.J.; Corcoran, S.L.; Ramulu, P.Y. Use of various glaucoma surgeries and procedures in Medicare beneficiaries from 1994 to 2012. *Ophthalmology* **2015**, *122*, 1615–1624.
8. Byun, Y.S.; Lee, N.Y.; Park, C.K. Risk factors of implant exposure outside the conjunctiva after Ahmed glaucoma valve implantation. *Jpn. J. Ophthalmol.* **2009**, *53*, 114–119.
9. Allingham, R.R.; Moroi, S.; Shields, M.B.; Damji, K. *Shields' Textbook of Glaucoma*; Lippincott Williams & Wilkins: Baltimore, MD, USA, 2020.
10. Koo, E.B.; Hou, J.; Han, Y.; Keenan, J.D.; Stamper, R.L.; Jeng, B.H. Effect of glaucoma tube shunt parameters on cornea endothelial cells in patients with Ahmed valve implants. *Cornea* **2015**, *34*, 37–41.

11. Tan, A.N.; Webers, C.A.; Berendschot, T.T.; de Brabander, J.; de Witte, P.M.; Nuijts, R.M.; Schouten, J.S.; Beckers, H.J. Corneal endothelial cell loss after Baerveldt glaucoma drainage device implantation in the anterior chamber. *Acta Ophthalmol.* **2017**, *95*, 91–96.
12. Lee, H.M.; Kim, K.N.; Park, K.S.; Lee, N.H.; Lee, S.B.; Kim, C.-S. Relationship between Tube Parameters and Corneal Endothelial Cell Damage after Ahmed Glaucoma Valve Implantation: A Comparative Study. *J. Clin. Med.* **2020**, *9*, 2546.
13. Poinoosawmy, D.; Nagasubramanian, S.; Brown, N. Effect of pilocarpine on visual acuity and on the dimensions of the cornea and anterior chamber. *Br. J. Ophthalmol.* **1976**, *60*, 676–679.
14. Abramson, D.H.; Coleman, D.J.; Forbes, M.; Franzen, L.A. Pilocarpine: Effect on the anterior chamber and lens thickness. *Arch. Ophthalmol.* **1972**, *87*, 615–620.
15. Koeppl, C.; Findl, O.; Menapace, R.; Kriechbaum, K.; Wirtitsch, M.; Buehl, W.; Sacu, S.; Drexler, W. Pilocarpine-induced shift of an accommodating intraocular lens: AT-45 Crystalens. *J. Cataract Refract. Surg.* **2005**, *31*, 1290–1297.
16. Langenbucher, A.; Seitz, B.; Huber, S.; Nguyen, N.X.; Küchle, M. Theoretical and measured pseudophakic accommodation after implantation of a new accommodative posterior chamber intraocular lens. *Arch. Ophthalmol.* **2003**, *121*, 1722–1727.
17. Kriechbaum, K.; Findl, O.; Koeppl, C.; Menapace, R.; Drexler, W. Stimulus-driven versus pilocarpine-induced biometric changes in pseudophakic eyes. *Ophthalmology* **2005**, *112*, 453–459.
18. Lea, S.H.; Rubinstein, M.; Snead, M.; Haworth, S. Pseudophakic accommodation? A study of the stability of capsular bag supported, one piece, rigid tripod, or soft flexible implants. *Br. J. Ophthalmol.* **1990**, *74*, 22–25.
19. Findl, O.; Kiss, B.; Petternel, V.; Menapace, R.; Georgopoulos, M.; Rainer, G.; Drexler, W. Intraocular lens movement caused by ciliary muscle contraction. *J. Cataract Refract. Surg.* **2003**, *29*, 669–676.
20. Vinod, K.; Gedde, S.J.; Feuer, W.J.; Panarelli, J.F.; Chang, T.C.; Chen, P.P.; Parrish, R.K. Practice preferences for glaucoma surgery: A survey of the American Glaucoma Society. *J. Glaucoma* **2017**, *26*, 687.
21. Hau, S.; Scott, A.; Bunce, C.; Barton, K. Corneal endothelial morphology in eyes implanted with anterior chamber aqueous shunts. *Cornea* **2011**, *30*, 50–55.
22. Kim, J.-H.; Kim, C.-S. The change in corneal endothelial cells after ahmed glaucoma valve implantation. *J. Korean Ophthalmol. Soc.* **2006**, *47*, 1972–1980.
23. Lee, E.-K.; Yun, Y.-J.; Lee, J.-E.; Yim, J.-H.; Kim, C.-S. Changes in corneal endothelial cells after Ahmed glaucoma valve implantation: 2-year follow-up. *Am. J. Ophthalmol.* **2009**, *148*, 361–367.
24. Park, H.L.; Jung, K.; Park, C. Serial intracameral visualization of the Ahmed glaucoma valve tube by anterior segment optical coherence tomography. *Eye* **2012**, *26*, 1256–1262.
25. Seo, J.W.; Lee, J.Y.; Nam, D.H.; Lee, D.Y. Comparison of the changes in corneal endothelial cells after pars plana and anterior chamber ahmed valve implant. *J. Ophthalmol.* **2015**, *2015*, 486832.
26. Gandham, S.B.; Costa, V.P.; Katz, L.J.; Wilson, R.P.; Sivalingam, A.; Belmont, J.; Smith, M. Aqueous tube-shunt implantation and pars plana vitrectomy in eyes with refractory glaucoma. *Am. J. Ophthalmol.* **1993**, *116*, 189–195.
27. Faghihi, H.; Hajizadeh, F.; Mohammadi, S.F.; Kadkhoda, A.; Peyman, G.A.; Riazi-Esfahani, M. Pars plana Ahmed valve implant and vitrectomy in the management of neovascular glaucoma. *Ophthalmic Surg. Lasers Imaging Retin.* **2007**, *38*, 292–300.
28. Weiner, A.; Cohn, A.D.; Balasubramaniam, M.; Weiner, A.J. Glaucoma tube shunt implantation through the ciliary sulcus in pseudophakic eyes with high risk of corneal decompensation. *J. Glaucoma* **2010**, *19*, 405–411.
29. Eslami, Y.; Mohammadi, M.; Fakhraie, G.; Zarei, R.; Moghimi, S. Ahmed glaucoma valve implantation with tube insertion through the ciliary sulcus in pseudophakic/aphakic eyes. *J. Glaucoma* **2014**, *23*, 115–118.
30. Drugs.com. Available online: https://www.drugs.com/ppa/pilocarpine-ophthalmic.html (accessed on 17 August 2020).
31. Rękas, M.; Barchan-Kucia, K.; Konopińska, J.; Mariak, Z.; Żarnowski, T. Analysis and modeling of anatomical changes of the anterior segment of the eye after cataract surgery with consideration of different phenotypes of eye structure. *Curr. Eye Res.* **2015**, *40*, 1018–1027.
32. Olsen, T. Prediction of the effective postoperative (intraocular lens) anterior chamber depth. *J. Cataract Refract. Surg.* **2006**, *32*, 419–424.
33. Memarzadeh, F.; Tang, M.; Li, Y.; Chopra, V.; Francis, B.A.; Huang, D. Optical coherence tomography assessment of angle anatomy changes after cataract surgery. *Am. J. Ophthalmol.* **2007**, *144*, 464–465.
34. Shin, H.C.; Subrayan, V.; Tajunisah, I. Changes in anterior chamber depth and intraocular pressure after phacoemulsification in eyes with occludable angles. *J. Cataract Refract. Surg.* **2010**, *36*, 1289–1295.
35. Altan, C.; Bayraktar, S.; Altan, T.; Eren, H.; Yilmaz, O.F. Anterior chamber depth, iridocorneal angle width, and intraocular pressure changes after uneventful phacoemulsification in eyes without glaucoma and with open iridocorneal angles. *J. Cataract Refract. Surg.* **2004**, *30*, 832–838.
36. Huang, G.; Gonzalez, E.; Peng, P.-H.; Lee, R.; Leeungurasatien, T.; He, M.; Porco, T.; Lin, S.C. Anterior chamber depth, iridocorneal angle width, and intraocular pressure changes after phacoemulsification: Narrow vs open iridocorneal angles. *Arch. Ophthalmol.* **2011**, *129*, 1283–1290.

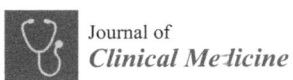

Article

Outcomes of Small Size Ahmed Glaucoma Valve Implantation in Asian Chronic Angle-Closure Glaucoma

Ke-Hao Huang [1,2], Ching-Long Chen [1], Da-Wen Lu [1], Jiann-Torng Chen [1] and Yi-Hao Chen [1,*]

1. Department of Ophthalmology, Tri-Service General Hospital, National Defense Medical Center, Taipei 114, Taiwan; a912572000@gmail.com (K.-H.H.); doc30881@mail.ndmctsgh.edu.tw (C-L.C.); ludawen@yahoo.com (D.-W.L.); jt66chen@gmail.com (J.-T.C.)
2. Department of Ophthalmology, Song-Shan Branch of Tri-Service General Hospital, National Defense Medical Center, Taipei 105, Taiwan
* Correspondence: doc30879@mail.ndmctsgh.edu.tw; Tel.: +886-2-8792-7163

Abstract: For chronic angle-closure glaucoma (ACG), Ahmed glaucoma valve (AGV) is a useful drainage device for intraocular pressure (IOP) control but there are few reports discussing the outcomes of small size AGV in adult patients. This retrospective study involved 43 Asian adult patients (43 eyes) with chronic ACG. All patients had undergone small size AGV insertion and were divided into anterior chamber (AC) group and posterior chamber (PC) group. In the AC group, tube was inserted through sclerectomy gap into the anterior chamber. In the PC group, tube was inserted into posterior chamber through a needling tract. Outcome measures were intraocular pressure (IOP), visual acuity, number of antiglaucoma medications, survival curve and incidence of complications. In total, 43 eyes of 43 patients, 24 in the AC group and 19 in the PC group, were reviewed. The mean follow-up period was 28.5 months (95% confidence interval: 25.5–31.4). Mean IOP had significantly decreased following AGV insertion. The Kaplan–Meier survival analysis demonstrated a probability of success at 24 months of 67.4% for qualified success and 39.5% for complete success. There were no significant differences between the AC and PC groups in terms of the mean IOP, cumulative probability of success, visual acuity change or antiglaucoma medication change, except IOP at 1-day and 1-month mean IOP. The most common complications noted was hyphema in the PC group. For adult chronic ACG patients, small size AGV insertion could be effective at lowering IOP. Besides, tube insertion into AC with sclerectomy may prevent the hypertensive phase in the early postoperative period.

Keywords: Ahmed glaucoma valve; angle closure glaucoma; surgical modification; surgical outcome

Citation: Huang, K.-H.; Chen, C.-L.; Lu, D.-W.; Chen, J.-T.; Chen, Y.-H. Outcomes of Small Size Ahmed Glaucoma Valve Implantation in Asian Chronic Angle-Closure Glaucoma. *J. Clin. Med.* **2021**, *10*, 813. https://doi.org/10.3390/jcm10040813

Academic Editor: Georgios Labiris

Received: 4 February 2021
Accepted: 15 February 2021
Published: 17 February 2021

Publisher's Note: MDPI stays neutral with regard to jurisdictional claims in published maps and institutional affiliations.

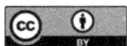

Copyright: © 2021 by the authors. Licensee MDPI, Basel, Switzerland. This article is an open access article distributed under the terms and conditions of the Creative Commons Attribution (CC BY) license (https://creativecommons.org/licenses/by/4.0/).

1. Introduction

Angle closure glaucoma (ACG) is caused by impaired outflow facility secondary to appositional or synechial closure of the anterior chamber drainage angle, which leads to elevated intraocular pressure (IOP), optic nerve damage and visual field loss. Based on etiology, ACG can be divided into primary or secondary ACG. In Asian populations, primary ACG is estimated to pose a greater risk of blindness than primary open-angle glaucoma [1]. The gold standard to treat ACG is reducing IOP by medication, peripheral iridotomy and controlling the underlying causes. However, some eyes are resistant to these treatments and thus surgical intervention may be necessary. Several surgical procedures, such as anterior chamber paracentesis, surgical iridectomy, simple lens extraction, trabeculectomy or a combination of lens extraction and trabeculectomy are utilized for treating ACG and different procedures are chosen according to patient's condition.

Implantation of Ahmed glaucoma valve (AGV) is effective to control IOP in glaucoma patients and there are two different size models for adult and children, respectively. The difference is the surface area, which is 184 mm^2 for adult and 96 mm^2 for children. AGV is indicated commonly for the patients who had failed previous trabeculectomy. In such cases, the availability of viable conjunctiva would be reduced and the risk of complications like conjunctival buttonhole, wound leak and tube or plate exposure may increase. In glaucoma patients with failed previous trabeculectomy, small size AGV may be beneficial to make AGV implantation possible because it can reduce the need of viable conjunctiva during surgery. Besides, data on AGV insertion in ACG are limited because of the relative high risk of corneal complications such as shallow anterior chamber and tube-corneal touch [2,3]. Previously, tube insertion via the ciliary sulcus or pars plana was reported to avoid these complications [4,5] but this technique cannot be performed easily and was not applicable in all cases of ACG. Therefore, evaluation of the outcomes of small size AGV in adult chronic ACG patients may provide useful information.

In the present study, we reported the results of small size AGV insertion in adult chronic ACG patients. And we also evaluated the benefit and safety of modified technique (sclerectomy) for AGV tube insertion to anterior chamber.

2. Materials and Methods

2.1. Patients

This retrospective review was carried out at a tertiary referral medical center in northern Taiwan between 2009 and 2014. The study was approved by the institutional review board of Tri-Service General Hospital, Taipei, Taiwan (TSGHIRB No. 1-103-05-144), which waived the requirement for informed consent from participants and allowed access to the follow-up clinical records. It was conducted in accordance with the requirements of the Declaration of Helsinki. Patients with chronic ACG with an uncontrolled IOP who had undergone a small size AGV insertion were included. Chronic ACG was defined by the following criteria: patients had surgical history of previously failed trabeculectomy and the angle presentation of the eye was lower than grade 2 before surgery, according to the Shaffer gonioscopic grading system and with glaucomatous changes including abnormal optic disc appearance, loss of the nerve fiber layer and visual field defects. Uncontrolled IOP was defined as an IOP > 21 mmHg, even after maximal usage of antiglaucoma medications. Exclusion criteria included primary angle-closure suspect, primary angle closure with no optic nerve damage, any ocular surgeries within the previous 3 months, a follow-up period less than 2 years, a preoperative visual acuity (VA) lower than light perception or were younger than 20 years of age. Besides, the decision of small size AGV implantation is made by surgeon during surgery, based on the conjunctival mobility, scarring due to previous surgery like trabeculectomy and limited surgical area which may be due to conjunctival scarring or small fissure height that even the maximum extension is made by lid speculum and traction suture. This study enrolled 46 chronic ACG patients. 3 of them were lost to follow up and were excluded from the analysis. In the remaining 43 patients, 24 patients were in the anterior chamber (AC) group and the other 19 patients were in the posterior chamber (PC) group, which was based on the presence of anterior synechiae at tube insertion site or not.

Patients' demographic characteristics, namely best-refracted VA, IOP, number of antiglaucoma medications, type of chronic ACG and history of ocular surgery, systemic diseases or complications were recorded and assessed by a chart review. VA was measured via a standard Snellen chart and IOP via the Goldmann applanation tonometer. Defining the time of operation as the baseline, each patient was followed up 1 day, 2 weeks, 1 month, 3 months, 6 months, 1 year, 2 years and 3 years after surgery.

2.2. Outcome Measures

Mean IOP, vision changes, complications and the number of antiglaucoma medications taken after the Ahmed glaucoma valve insertion were evaluated as the outcome measures. Qualified success was defined by an IOP < 21 mmHg with or without antiglaucoma medications; complete success was defined by an IOP < 21 mmHg without additional therapy; failure was defined by (1) an IOP > 21 mmHg despite the use of antiglaucoma medications at 2 consecutive visits, (2) light perception negative vision, (3) requirement of additional glaucoma surgery or (4) devastating operative or postoperative complications such as endophthalmitis or phthisis.

2.3. Surgical Technique

Surgical and postoperative management procedures were similar across all patients and the procedures were shown in Figure 1.

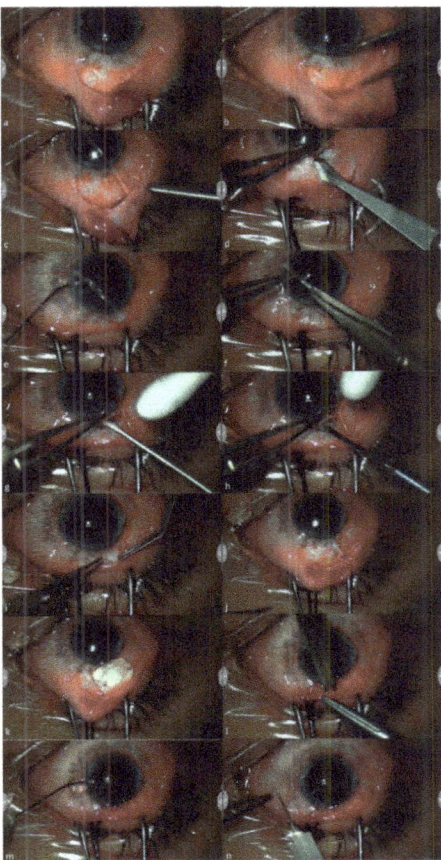

Figure 1. Surgical technique description. (**a**) fornix-based conjunctival flap was created in the superotemporal quadrant between two adjacent recti muscles under general anesthesia. (**b**) Ahmed plate would be placed 7 mm posterior to the corneoscleral limbus. (**c**) Ahmed plate is fixed firmly to the sclera with 8-0 prolene sutures. (**d**). 6 mm limbus-based triangular partial thickness scleral flap was created. (**e**) anterior chamber paracentesis was made by microvitreoretinal (MVR) blade and viscoelastic was injected through the paracentesis. (**f**) the tube was trimmed. (**g**) anterior chamber incision at limbus was made by MVR blade. (**h**) sclerectomy gap was made by Kelly Descemet's membrane punch. (**i**) the residual length of tube was modified as desired (about 1–2 mm in anterior chamber). (**j**) the scleral flap was closed with 10-0 nylon sutures and the tube was secured with 8–0 prolene suture. (**k**) A human donor scleral graft was placed on the tube with the anterior edge adjacent to the limbus and sutured to the sclera with an 8-0 Vicryl suture. (**l**) The conjunctiva was then re-approximated with 8-0 Vicryl interrupted sutures. (**m**) viscoelastic anterior chamber injection was repeated to avoid early postoperative hypotony. (**n**) subconjunctival injection of dexamethasone and gentamicin.

In each case, a fornix-based conjunctival flap was created in the superotemporal or superonasal quadrant between two adjacent recti muscles under general anesthesia. The AGV (model S3 or FP-8, New World Medical, Rancho Cucamonga, CA, USA) was irrigated with balanced saline solution (BSS, Alcon, Fort Worth, TX, USA) to prime the valve mechanism. The plate was soaked with 0.4 mg/mL mitomycin-C and then was wiped dry 10 s later. And it was placed at least 7 mm posterior to the corneoscleral limbus and fixed firmly to the sclera with 8-0 prolene sutures (Ethicon Inc., Somerville, NJ, USA). A 6 mm limbus-based triangular partial thickness scleral flap was created at the site of tube incision. Anterior chamber paracentesis was made by microvitreoretinal (MVR) blade and about 0.1 mL viscoelastic (Healon GV, Advanced Medical Optics, Santa Ana, CA, USA) injection was performed through the paracentesis. The tube was trimmed and the residual length was left as desired.

In AC group, anterior chamber incision was made by MVR blade under the scleral flap through the limbus and then a sclerectomy gap was made by Kelly Descemet's membrane punch. The tube in the anterior chamber was left a length of 1–2 mm lying on the iris and away from the corneal endothelium.

The decision of tube insertion to AC or PC is based on the condition of the tube insertion site. If there were possible complications for AC insertion like tube–endothelial contact, patients with anterior synechiae at tube insertion site would be arranged to PC group. In PC group, the tube was inserted to ciliary sulcus (1.5 mm posterior to the limbus) through a tract which is made by 23 G needle without sclerectomy. It is not possible to perform sclerectomy in PC group due to the anatomical consideration, which ciliary body could be damaged after sclerectomy. The difference between AC and PC group was shown in Figure 2.

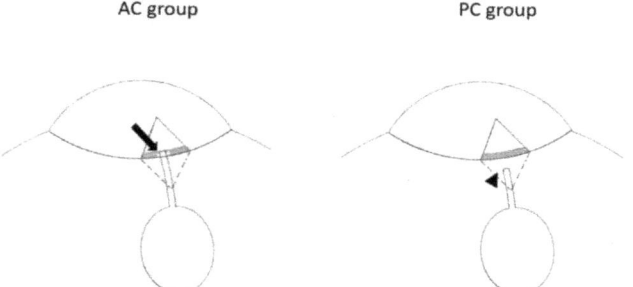

Figure 2. The difference between anterior chamber (AC) group and posterior chamber (PC) group. In the AC group, the tube was inserted into anterior chamber through the sclerectomy gap (arrow) under partial thickness scleral flap. In the PC group, the tube was inserted to ciliary sulcus (arrowhead; 1.5 mm posterior to the limbus) through 23 G needling tract.

After the tube was inserted, the superficial scleral flap was closed tightly with 10-0 nylon sutures (Ethicon Inc., Somerville, NJ, USA). And the tube was secured with 8-0 prolene suture. A human donor scleral graft was placed on the tube with the anterior edge adjacent to the limbus and sutured to the sclera with an 8-0 Vicryl suture (Ethicon Inc., Somerville, NJ, USA). The conjunctiva was then re-approximated with 8-0 Vicryl interrupted sutures. And then 0.2 mL viscoelastic anterior chamber injection was repeated to avoid early postoperative hypotony. In the end of the surgery, a subconjunctival injection of dexamethasone and gentamicin was administered.

All surgeries were performed by the authors, DW Lu and YH Chen. After the operation, topical antibiotic (tobramycin or norfloxacin) and steroid (prednisolone acetate) eye drops were applied routinely for 4–8 weeks and tapered gradually. Viscoelastic anterior chamber reformation was performed under a slit-lamp if early flat chamber was noted after surgery. Antiglaucoma medications were adjusted based on IOP and the clinical status of the operated eye.

2.4. Statistical Methods

All data are presented as mean (95% confidence interval (CI)). The distributions of variables in the 2 groups were compared using the unpaired Student's t test for continuous variables and the chi-square or Fisher exact test for categorical data. IOP values were compared by the Wilcoxon signed-rank test or Mann-Whitney U test. In addition, post-hoc power was calculated if significant IOP difference was noted assuming a two-sided alpha = 0.05 for the fixed sample size ($n = 43$) of the present study. A Kaplan-Meier life table analysis was conducted to access the survival rates of the surgical method. $p < 0.05$ was considered statistically significant. All statistical analyses were performed using GraphPad Prism 5.0 (GraphPad Software, Inc, San Diego, CA, USA).

3. Results

In total, 43 patients with chronic ACG were included in this study: 24 patients in the AC group and 19 in the PC group. The demographic characteristics of the total patient population and of the AC and PC groups are shown in Table 1. Twenty-four eyes had undergone prior trabeculectomies and twenty eyes had undergone prior cataract surgeries in the AC group; all eyes had undergone prior trabeculectomies and cataract surgeries in the PC group. All included patients did not have surgical history of vitrectomy. The mean follow-up time of all patients were 29.5 months (95% CI: 24.8–34.2) for the AC group and 27.2 months (95% CI: 23.5–30.8) for the PC group.

Table 1. Demographic Characteristics of the Patient Cohort.

	AC Group ($n = 24$)	PC Group ($n = 19$)	p
Age (Years)	54.7 (95% CI: 48.7–60.6)	58.8 (95% CI: 51.8–65.8)	0.2397
Sex			
Male	8	10	0.2304
Female	16	9	
Eye			
Right	12	6	0.3510
Left	12	13	
Lens status			
Phakic	4	0	0.1175
Pseudophakic	20	19	
Mean pre-operative intraocular pressure (mmHg)	36.8 (95% CI: 32.4–41.1)	42.2 (95% CI: 37.2–47.2)	0.1036
Mean pre-operative glaucoma medications	2.7 (95% CI: 2.4–3.0)	3.1 (95% CI: 2.8–3.5)	0.0811
Previous surgery			
Trabeculectomy	24	19	
Cataract surgery	20	19	0.1175
Vitrectomy	0	0	
Disease type			
PACG	10	4	0.5623

Table 1. Cont.

	AC Group (n = 24)	PC Group (n = 19)	p
UG	3	4	
NVG	6	4	
PKG	4	6	
Other	1	1	
Follow-up (Months)	29.5 (95% CI: 24.8–34.2)	27.2 (95% CI: 23.5–30.8)	0.4350

PACG = primary angle closure glaucoma; UG = uveitic glaucoma; NVG = neovascular glaucoma; PKG = post keratoplasty glaucoma; AC: anterior chamber; PC: posterior chamber; CI: confidence interval.

Table 2 represents mean IOP data for all patients, not only successful but also failed patients' IOP data were collected at all time intervals since preoperative to postoperative follow-up period. Compared with the baseline value, IOP differed significantly over time ($p < 0.05$) in the total patient population and in both the AC and PC groups. There were no significant differences between the AC and PC groups at any of the time points except at 1-day ($p = 0.0160$) and 1-month ($p < 0.0001$) post-surgery. The mean IOP at 1-day and 1-month post-surgery was 8.5 mmHg (95% CI: 7.6–9.4) and 12.1 mmHg (95% CI: 11.2–13.1) in the AC group and 10.6 mmHg (95% CI: 9.3–11.9) and 20.0 mmHg (95% CI: 17.0–23.0) in the PC group, respectively. As shown in Figure 3, IOP was noted to be significantly higher in the PC group than in the AC group at 1-day and 1-month post-surgery. Post-hoc statistical power for detecting the IOP difference was 76.8% for 1-day IOP and 99.9% for 1-month IOP.

Table 2. Mean Intraocular Pressures (IOP) of the Patient Cohort (mmHg).

	Total (n = 43)	AC Group (n = 24)	PC Group (n = 19)	p
Preoperative (Day 0)	39.2 (95% CI: 35.9–42.4)	36.8 (95% CI: 32.4–41.1)	42.2 (95% CI: 37.2–47.2)	0.1036
First day (Day 1)	9.4 (95% CI: 8.6–10.2)	8.5 (95% CI: 7.6–9.4)	10.6 (95% CI: 9.3–11.9)	0.0160 *
Seventh day (Day 7)	12.1 (95% CI: 10.9–13.3)	12.5 (95% CI: 10.9–14.2)	11.6 (95% CI: 9.72–13.4)	0.5067
First month (Day 30)	15.6 (95% CI: 13.8–17.4)	12.1 (95% CI: 11.2–13.1)	20.0 (95% CI: 17.0–23.0)	<0.0001 *
Third month (Day 90)	16.1 (95% CI: 14.3–17.8)	15.6 (95% CI: 12.8–17.5)	17.2 (95% CI: 14.4–20.0)	0.1135
Sixth month (Day 180)	15.7 (95% CI: 14.9–16.6)	15.5 (95% CI: 14.4–16.6)	16.1 (95% CI: 14.7–17.4)	0.7197
First year (Day 360)	19.0 (95% CI: 17.6–20.3)	19.6 (95% CI: 17.5–21.7)	18.1 (95% CI: 16.5–19.7)	0.5049
Second year (Day 720)	20.2 (95% CI: 17.8–22.5)	19.5 (95% CI: 16.5–22.5)	21.1 (95% CI: 17.1–25.2)	0.5236

Addressed IOP data includes successful and failed patients. AC: anterior chamber; PC: posterior chamber; CI: confidence interval.
*: $p < 0.05$.

The Kaplan-Meier survival curves for qualified success of the total patient population and the AC and PC groups are shown in Figure 4A. The probability of qualified success was 67.4% at 24 months for all patients (AC group versus PC group: 70.8% versus 63.2%). No significant differences ($p = 0.67$, log rank test) were noted between the AC and PC groups. Of the 7 failed eyes in the AC group, 5 underwent second AGV insertions, 1 underwent evisceration of the eyeball and 1 underwent a cyclodestructive procedure. Of the 7 failed eyes in the PC group, 5 underwent second AGV implantations and 2 underwent cyclodestructive procedures. When complete success was used as the criterion, the Kaplan-Meier survival curves for the total patient population and the AC and PC groups are shown in Figure 4B. The probability of complete success was 39.5% at 24 months for all patients (AC group versus PC group: 45.8% versus 31.6%). There were no significant differences ($p = 0.43$, log rank test) between the AC and PC groups.

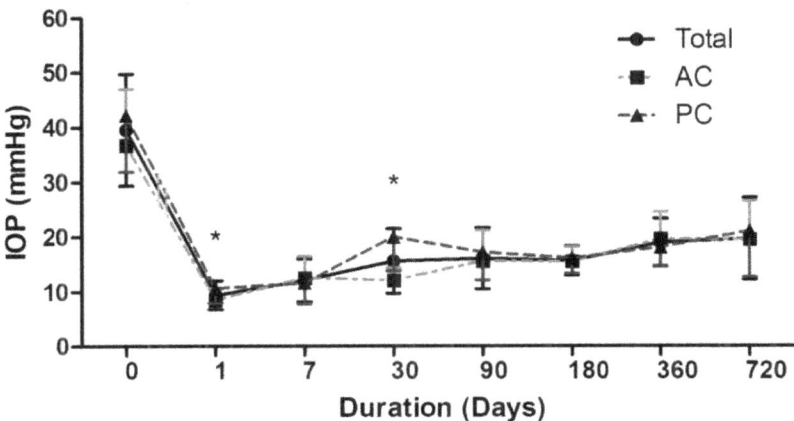

Figure 3. Preoperative and postoperative intraocular pressure (IOP) after Ahmed glaucoma valve implantation surgery plotted over time. Addressed IOP data includes successful and failed patients. AC: anterior chamber; PC: posterior chamber. *: $p < 0.05$.

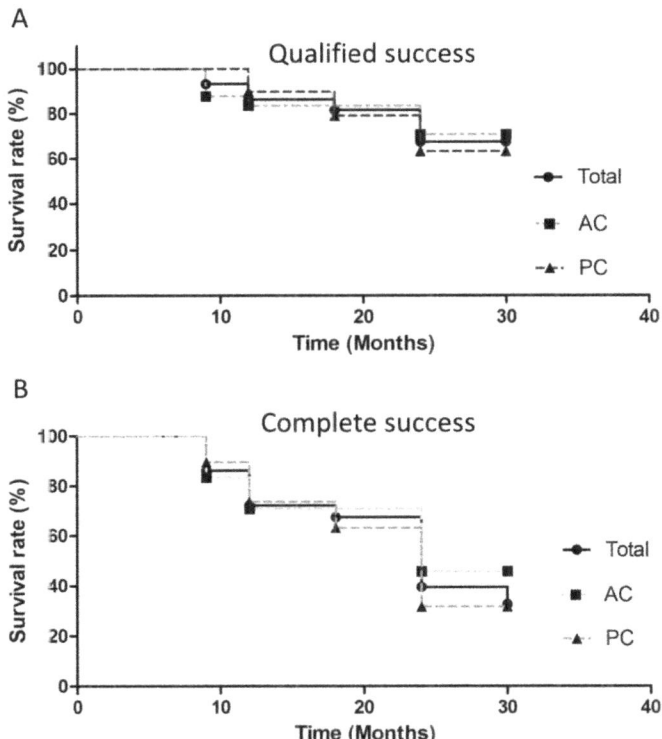

Figure 4. Kaplan-Meier curve showing the probability of qualified success (**A**) ($p = 0.67$, log rank test for comparing AC and PC surviving curves) and complete success (**B**) ($p = 0.43$, log rank test for comparing AC and PC surviving curves) after Ahmed glaucoma valve implantation surgery. AC: anterior chamber; PC: posterior chamber.

A comparison of the final changes in the vision of the total patient population and both the AC and PC groups is shown in Figure 5A. There were no significant differences between the AC and PC groups with respect to "worse," "better" or "no change" classifications. In the AC group, 12 patients (50%) showed no change in vision, 4 (16.7%) showed an improvement and 8 (33.3%) showed a decline. Similarly, 11 patients in the PC group (57.9%) showed no change in vision, 3 (15.8%) showed an improvement and 5 (26.3%) showed a decline (Table 3).

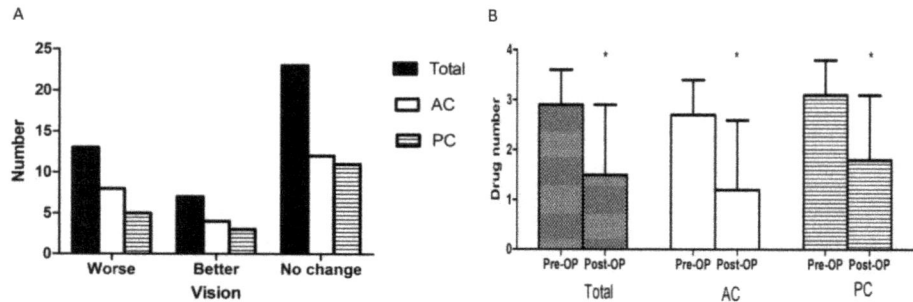

Figure 5. Changes in vision (A) and number of antiglaucoma medications (B) between the baseline and the final visit. AC: anterior chamber; PC: posterior chamber; OP: operation. *: $p < 0.05$.

Table 3. Final Vision Changes of the Patient Cohort

	Total (n = 43)	AC Group (n = 24)	PC Group (n = 19)	p
Worse	13	8	5	0.8601
Better	7	4	3	
No change	23	12	11	

AC: anterior chamber; PC: posterior chamber.

In terms of changes in antiglaucoma medication, the number of antiglaucoma drugs used preoperatively and postoperatively are shown in Figure 5B. In the total patient population and both the AC and PC groups, significant differences were noted between the number of preoperative and postoperative medications (Table 4). The average number of antiglaucoma medications used prior to AGV implantation was 2.7 (95% CI: 2.4–3.0) in the AC group and 3.1 (95% CI: 2.8–3.5) in the PC group. This difference between the two groups was not statistically significant. After AGV implantation, the mean number of medications used was 1.2 (95% CI: 0.6–1.8) in the AC group and 1.8 (95% CI: 1.2–2.5) in the PC group. This difference between the two groups was also not statistically significant.

Table 4. Mean Number of Antiglaucoma Medications of the Patient Cohort.

	Preoperative	Postoperative	p
Total (n = 43)	2.9 (95% CI: 2.7–3.1)	1.5 (95% CI: 1.0–1.9)	<0.0001 *
AC group (n = 24)	2.7 (95% CI: 2.4–3.0)	1.2 (95% CI: 0.6–1.8)	<0.0001 *
PC group (n = 19)	3.1 (95% CI: 2.8–3.5)	1.8 (95% CI: 1.2–2.5)	0.0024 *

AC: anterior chamber; PC: posterior chamber; CI: confidence interval. *: $p < 0.05$.

No intraoperative complications were noted in this study and the postoperative complications are listed in Table 5. The early postoperative complications occurring in the first month were hyphema, flat chamber/hypotony and tube or plate exposure. The frequency of hyphema was significantly higher in the PC group than in the AC group ($p < 0.05$) and this complication was resolved spontaneously. Although there was no statistically significant difference in the complication of flat chamber/hypotony, a higher incidence of viscoelastic anterior chamber reformation was 0.5 more in the AC group (0.9 ± 0.7 vs. 0.4 ± 0.8; $p < 0.05$). The late postoperative complications, which occurred more than 3 months post-surgery, were tube retraction, encapsulated bleb, endophthalmitis, bullous keratopathy and strabismus. There were no significant differences between the AC and PC groups with respect to these late complications. More than one complication was noted in some eyes.

Table 5. Post-operative Complications in the Patient Cohort.

	Total (n, %)	AC Group (n, %)	PC Group (n, %)	p
Hyphema	6, 14.0%	1, 4.2%	5, 26.3%	0.0374 *
Flat chamber/Hypotony	2, 4.7%	1, 4.2%	1, 5.3%	0.8654
Tube or plate exposure	2, 4.7%	1, 4.2%	1, 5.3%	0.8654
Tube retraction	3, 7.0%	1, 4.2%	2, 10.5%	0.4163
Encapsulated bleb	6, 14.0%	3, 12.5%	3, 15.8%	0.7572
Endophthalmitis	1, 2.3%	1, 4.2%	0, 0%	0.3680
Bullous keratopathy	3, 7.0%	2, 8.3%	1, 5.3%	0.6947
Strabismus	0, 0%	0, 0%	0, 0%	

AC: anterior chamber; PC: posterior chamber. *: $p < 0.05$.

4. Discussion

ACG accounts for a large proportion of glaucoma cases in Asia [6] and needs to be adequately managed. The strategy for treating ACG is releasing the pupillary block using laser peripheral iridotomy and maintain IOP with or without medication. Glaucoma surgery is performed to lower IOP when further IOP reduction cannot be achieved by medical or laser treatment. The implantation of a glaucoma drainage device is one surgical option. One example of such a device is an AGV, which consists of a flow resistance valve. AGV insertion has been reported in uveitic and pediatric glaucoma with varying results [7,8]. In past reports, mean IOP was maintained below the teens and the cumulative probability of success was 68–75% at 2 years after AGV implantation [3,9]. Our results were similar to those of previous studies: mean IOP decreased to 9.4 mmHg at day 1 and 20.2 mmHg at 2 years and the cumulative probability of qualified success was 67.4% at 2 years after AGV implantation. In most eyes (69.8%), Vision was maintained or improved after AGV implantation. The mean number of antiglaucoma medications also decreased from 2.9 to 1.5 after AGV implantation. Although the development of narrow angle in uveitic, neovascular or post-penetrating keratoplasty glaucoma is associated with poor prognosis with respect to IOP control, our study demonstrated that the results of AGV implantation in chronic ACG may not be inferior to the results in other glaucoma types.

Therapeutically, the success of IOP control after tube shunt surgery is related to the size of the plate, plate material, profile, surface texture and the severity of surgical damage [10]. IOP reduction is greater when a larger plate is used. However, in our study, the cumulative probability of success of AGV implantation was not inferior to other studies although we used the small size AGV. East Asian individuals are considered to have small eyes, puffy eyelids and shallow orbits [11,12]. Besides, in our study, all the included patients have some extent of conjunctival scarring and limited surgical view. In these individuals, therefore, implantation of adult-sized AGVs may be difficult to manipulate and may cause more complication like conjunctival buttonhole, wound leak and tube or plate exposure and strabismus. Small size AGV implantation may decrease tissue damage and then lower the severity of surgical trauma and scar formation in these patients. In our research, small size AGV implantation could also be effective at lowering IOP for Asian adult chronic

ACG patients, exhibiting an acceptable cumulative probability of success and less ocular tissue damage.

The conventional procedure of AGV implantation involves puncture of the anterior chamber by a needle for tube insertion. However, this is difficult in eyes with ACG because tube in shallow anterior chamber may damage adjacent tissues such as the cornea or iris. Therefore, AGV implantation is relatively contraindicated in ACG. To reduce this risk, tube insertion through the posterior chamber or pars plana has been reported. However, tube insertion through the posterior chamber cannot be performed in phakic eyes and insertion through the pars plana is a difficult technique. In this study, we used sclerectomy instead of needle puncture in the AC group and the sclerectomy gap could provide a larger space for tube insertion without injuring adjacent tissue. Moreover, we left a relative short length of the tube (1–2 mm) in the AC group. We believe that such modification could make the tube lie on the iris and reduce the chance of tube-endothelium contact, as shown in Figure 6. In our series, the incidence of bullous keratopathy did not differ between the AC and PC groups. The short tube length may result in tube retraction because of dynamic movement of the AGV tube with eye movement and such complication has previously been reported [13]. And tube retraction could lead to complete retraction from the anterior chamber. However, the frequency of tube retraction did not differ between both groups in our study, which may be due to the firm fixation of the AGV plate using a non-absorbable suture. In our study, tube insertion through sclerectomy gap and short tube length left in the AC group may be a safe procedure in eyes with chronic ACG.

The hypertensive phase is defined as a transient IOP elevation associated with an encapsulated bleb in the early postoperative period, which peaked in the first month and had stabilized by 6 months after the operation. The mechanism of hypertensive phase is presumably due to inflammatory mediators related congested, thickened, encapsulated bleb around the plate of the implant and cause increased resistance to aqueous flow. It has been reported to be more prevalent in eyes after AGV implantation [14,15], which may be related to the plate surface, the biomaterial or the absence of tube ligation. Pakravan [16] reported that early aqueous suppressant treatment in AGV implantation could reduce hypertensive phase frequency, which may be due to a lower concentration of inflammatory mediators reaching the tissues surrounding the AGV plate. In our study, mean IOP elevated in the PC group at 1 month, representing the hypertensive phase. In contrast, no such elevation was observed in the AC group. We believe such difference is because of sclerectomy. In the PC group, the aqueous humor accompanied with inflammatory mediators would be drained to the area around AGV plate directly and resulted in hypertensive phase. And such condition may not happen in the AC group because the aqueous humor could be drained through sclerectomy gap to peri-limbal area instead of posterior conjunctiva around AGV plate. Moreover, the sclerectomy gap could control IOP via the filtering function at the early postoperative period. Consistent with the previous theory [16], a lower concentration of inflammatory mediators around AGV plate may led to a thinner and looser Tenon's capsule, accounting for the noted absence of a hypertensive phase in the AC group.

The most common early postoperative complication in our study was transient hyphema (14.0%), followed by flat chamber/hypotony (4.7%). In previous studies of glaucoma drainage devices, hyphema was reported in 13–16.9% [17,18] and shallow anterior chamber/hypotony in 3–32% of cases [2,3,8,18,19]. In our study, the higher rate of hyphema in the PC group may be explained by the blind puncture that we cannot observe the needling direction when puncturing the posterior chamber. Such blind puncture could result in iris or ciliary body trauma. In flat chamber/hypotony, there was no significant difference between both groups. However, the frequency of viscoelastic anterior chamber reformation was relative higher in the AC group (0.9 ± 0.7 in AC group vs. 0.4 ± 0.8 in PC group; $p < 0.05$). The higher rate of AC group reformation may be explained by sclerectomy gap, which could prevent hypertensive phase via the filtering function at the early postoperative period. However, the frequency of viscoelastic AC reformation is low and no severe complications like suprachoroidal effusion and suprachoroidal hemorrhage were noted in both groups. Thus, we believe that sclerectomy is a safe procedure for glaucoma surgeon. Fortunately, these two early complications (hyphema and flat chamber/hypotony) could be treated by closely observation and in-office procedure. Besides, two patients of tube/plate exposure were noted at the early following period and slit-lamp examination revealed unhealthy conjunctiva with pale appearance and sloughed conjunctival sutures. The possible reasons of such early post-operative period complication may be due to inadequate conjunctival sutures and poor conjunctival healing process. Fortunately, the conjunctiva of the two patients could be re-sutured under topical anesthesia. There was no significant difference in late complications or in the preoperative to postoperative change in vision between the two groups. In addition, postoperative strabismus was not observed in our study and we believe this is because small size AGV implantation prevented direct trauma to the extraocular muscle.

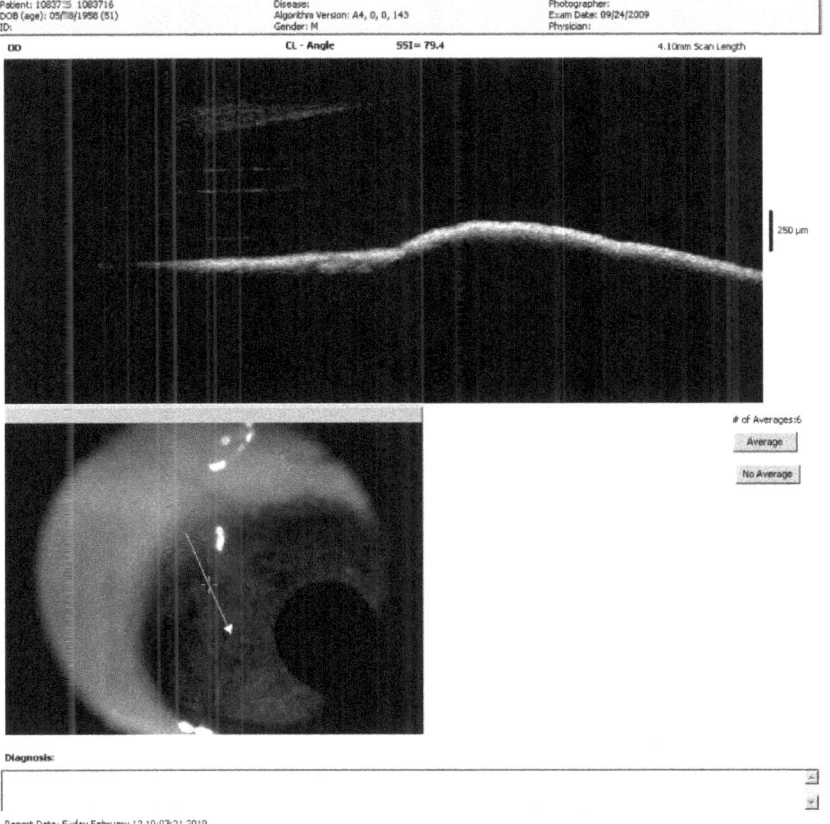

Figure 6. Image of sclerectomy-combined Ahmed glaucoma valve implantation into the anterior chamber by anterior optical coherence tomography, showing the tube lying on the iris.

There are some limitations to our study, including the small sample size, retrospective study design, heterogeneity of the study cohort, incomplete visual field data and the variability of follow-up periods. And the vision changes were established according to the patients' subjective responses, which could not quantify the vision changes. Besides, the decision of small size AGV was made by surgeon during surgery by the conjunctival scarring condition and surgical view, other objective parameters like axial length, orbital computed tomography (CT) to prove shallow orbit were not collected from the patients.

Above parameters may be considered in future prospective studies to provide more precise outcome. One important limitation is that all enrolled subjects in the present study were Asian, so the present results may not be applicable for other race.

5. Conclusions

In conclusion, in the 43 adult chronic adult ACG patients included in this study, small size AGV insertion showed an overall cumulative probability of success at 24 months were 67.4% for qualified success and 39.5% for complete success, indicating that small size AGV insertion could be effective at lowering IOP. Besides, tube insertion into anterior chamber with sclerectomy may prevent the hypertensive phase in the early postoperative period.

Author Contributions: Conceptualization, Y.-H.C. and D.-W.L.; methodology, Y.-H.C.; validation, Y.-H.C. and C.-L.C.; formal analysis, K.-H.H. and C.-L.C.; investigation, K.-H.H.; resources, D.-W.L. and Y.-H.C.; data curation, C.-L.C.; writing—original draft preparation, K.-H.H.; writing—review and editing, Y.-H.C. and D.-W.L.; supervision, D.-W.L. and J.-T.C. All authors have read and agreed to the published version of the manuscript.

Funding: This study was supported in by TSGH-D-110113 from the Tri-Service General Hospital and MOST-107-2314-B-016-032 from Ministry of Science and Technology.

Institutional Review Board Statement: The study was approved by the institutional review board of Tri-Service General Hospital, Taipei, Taiwan (TSGHIRB No. 1-103-05-144), which waived the requirement for informed consent from participants and allowed access to the follow-up clinical records. It was conducted in accordance with the requirements of the Declaration of Helsinki.

Informed Consent Statement: Patient consent was waived due to the retrospective type of this study, and the IRB waived the requirement for obtaining informed consent.

Data Availability Statement: The data presented in this study are available on reasonable request from the corresponding author.

Acknowledgments: The authors are thankful to Yu-Ching Chou, School of Public Health, National Defense Medical Center, Taipei, Taiwan for the statistical analysis.

Conflicts of Interest: The authors declare no conflict of interest.

References

1. Quigley, H.A.; Broman, A.T. The number of people with glaucoma worldwide in 2010 and 2020. *Br. J. Ophthalmol.* **2006**, *90*, 262–267. [CrossRef] [PubMed]
2. Coleman, A.L.; Hill, R.; Wilson, M.R.; Choplin, N.; Kotas-Neumann, R.; Tam, M.; Bacharach, J.; Panek, W.C. Initial Clinical Experience With the Ahmed Glaucoma Valve Implant. *Am. J. Ophthalmol.* **1995**, *120*, 23–31. [CrossRef]
3. Huang, M.C.; Netland, P.A.; Coleman, A.L.; Siegner, S.W.; Moster, M.R.; Hill, R.A. Intermediate-term clinical experience with the Ahmed Glaucoma Valve implant 1. *Am. J. Ophthalmol.* **1999**, *127*, 27–33. [CrossRef]
4. Sidoti, P.A.; Mosny, A.Y.; Ritterband, D.C.; Seedor, J.A. Pars plana tube insertion of glaucoma drainage implants and penetrating keratoplasty in patients with coexisting glaucoma and corneal disease. *Ophthalmology* **2001**, *108*, 1050–1058. [CrossRef]
5. Weiner, A.; Cohn, A.D.; Balasubramaniam, M.; Weiner, A.J. Glaucoma Tube Shunt Implantation Through the Ciliary Sulcus in Pseudophakic Eyes With High Risk of Corneal Decompensation. *J. Glaucoma* **2010**, *19*, 405–411. [CrossRef] [PubMed]
6. Yip, J.L.; Foster, P.J. Ethnic differences in primary angle-closure glaucoma. *Curr. Opin. Ophthalmol.* **2006**, *17*, 175–180. [CrossRef] [PubMed]
7. Da Mata, A.; Burk, S.E.; Netland, P.A.; Baltatzis, S.; Christen, W.; Foster, C.S. Management of uveitic glaucoma with Ahmed glaucoma valve implantation. *Ophthalmology* **1999**, *106*, 2168–2172. [CrossRef]
8. Englert, J.A.; Freedman, S.F.; Cox, T.A. The Ahmed valve in refractory pediatric glaucoma. *Am. J. Ophthalmol.* **1999**, *127*, 34–42. [CrossRef]
9. Topouzis, F.; Coleman, A.L.; Choplin, N.; Bethlem, M.M.; Hill, R.; Yu, F.; Panek, W.C.; Wilson, M. Follow-up of the original cohort with the Ahmed glaucoma valve implant 1. *Am. J. Ophthalmol.* **1999**, *128*, 198–204. [CrossRef]
10. Lim, K.S.; Allan, B.D.S.; Lloyd, A.W.; Muir, A.; Khaw, P.T. Glaucoma drainage devices; past, present, and future. *Br. J. Ophthalmol.* **1998**, *82*, 1083–1089. [CrossRef] [PubMed]
11. Kiranantawat, K.; Suhk, J.H.; Nguyen, A.H. The Asian Eyelid: Relevant Anatomy. *Semin. Plast. Surg.* **2015**, *29*, 158–164. [CrossRef] [PubMed]
12. Qin, B.; Tang, M.; Li, Y.; Zhang, X.; Chu, R.; Huang, D. Anterior Segment Dimensions in Asian and Caucasian Eyes Measured by Optical Coherence Tomography. *Ophthalmic Surg. Lasers Imaging* **2012**, *43*, 135–142. [CrossRef] [PubMed]

13. Park, H.-Y.L.; Jung, K.I.; Park, C.K. Serial intracameral visualization of the Ahmed glaucoma valve tube by anterior segment optical coherence tomography. *Eye* **2012**, *26*, 1256–1262. [CrossRef] [PubMed]
14. Ayyala, R.S.; Zurakowski, D.; Monshizadeh, R.; Hong, C.H.; Richards, D.; Layden, W.E.; Hutchinson, B.T.; Bellows, A.R. Comparison of double-plate Molteno and Ahmed glaucoma valve in patients with advanced uncontrolled glaucoma. *Ophthalmic Surg. Lasers* **2002**, *33*, 94–101. [PubMed]
15. Nouri-Mahdavi, K.; Caprioli, J. Evaluation of the hypertensive phase after insertion of the Ahmed Glaucoma Valve. *Am. J. Ophthalmol.* **2003**, *136*, 1001–1008. [CrossRef]
16. Pakravan, M.; Rad, S.S.; Yazdani, S.; Ghahari, E.; Yaseri, M. Effect of Early Treatment with Aqueous Suppressants on Ahmed Glaucoma Valve Implantation Outcomes. *Ophthalmology* **2014**, *121*, 1693–1698. [CrossRef] [PubMed]
17. Wilson, M.R.; Mendis, U.; Paliwal, A.; Haynatzka, V. Long-term follow-up of primary glaucoma surgery with Ahmed glaucoma valve implant versus trabeculectomy. *Am. J. Ophthalmol.* **2003**, *136*, 464–470. [CrossRef]
18. Budenz, D.L.; Barton, K.; Feuer, W.J.; Schiffman, J.; Costa, V.P.; Godfrey, D.G.; Buys, Y.M. Treatment Outcomes in the Ahmed Baerveldt Comparison Study after 1 Year of Follow-up. *Ophthalmology* **2011**, *118*, 443–452. [CrossRef] [PubMed]
19. Siegner, S.W.; Netland, P.A.; Urban, R.C., Jr.; Williams, A.S.; Richards, D.W.; Latina, M.A.; Brandt, J.D. Clinical Experience with the Baerveldt Glaucoma Drainage Implant. *Ophthalmology* **1995**, *102*, 1298–1307. [CrossRef]

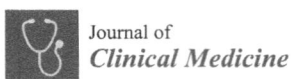

Article

The Effect of Antiglaucoma Procedures (Trabeculectomy vs. Ex-PRESS Glaucoma Drainage Implant) on the Corneal Biomechanical Properties

Aristeidis Konstantinidis *, Eirini-Kanella Panagiotopoulou, Georgios D. Panos, Haris Sideroudi, Aysel Mehmet and Georgios Labiris

Department of Ophthalmology, University Hospital of Alexandroupolis, 68131 Alexandroupolis, Greece; eipanagi@med.duth.gr (E.-K.P.); gdpanos@gmail.com (G.D.P.); hsideroudi@gmail.com (H.S.); ayselmehmet83@hotmail.com (A.M.); labiris@usa.net (G.L.)
* Correspondence: aristeidiskon@hotmail.com; Tel.: +30-694-669-6980

Abstract: The aim of this study is to investigate the effect of two antiglaucoma procedures, namely trabeculectomy and Ex-PRESS mini-shunt insertion on the biomechanical properties of the cornea. This is a prospective study. Thirty patients (30 eyes) were included in the study. Nineteen eyes had an Ex-PRESS shunt inserted (Group 1) and 11 had trabeculectomy (Group 2). The examination time points for both groups were one to three weeks preoperatively and at month 1, 6, and 12 postoperatively. Corneal biomechanical properties (corneal hysteresis (CH) corneal resistance factor (CRF)) were measured with the Ocular Response Analyzer (ORA). In group 1, CH was significantly increased at 6 and 12 months compared to baseline values. Corneal hysteresis was also higher at 1 month postoperatively, but this increase did not reach statistical significance. In group 2, the CH was significantly increased at all time points compared to the preoperative values. CRF decreased at all time points postoperatively compared to the preoperative values in both groups. The difference (preoperative values to postoperative values at all time points) of the CH and CRF between the two groups was also compared and no significant differences were detected between the two surgical techniques. Trabeculectomy and the EX-PRESS mini-shunt insertion significantly alter the corneal biomechanical properties as a result of the surgical trauma and the presence of the shunt in the corneal periphery. When compared between them, they affect the corneal biomechanical properties in a similar way.

Keywords: glaucoma; trabeculectomy; corneal hysteresis; corneal resistance factor

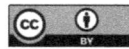

1. Introduction

Glaucoma is the second cause of blindness globally after cataract [1]. However unlike cataract it can cause irreversible loss of vision. Intraocular pressure (IOP) is a major risk factor for glaucomatous optic neuropathy and the only one that can be modified [2]. The initial treatment of the chronic forms of glaucoma is the conservative management with eye drops. In many cases, the drop of the IOP is not sufficient to slow down the optic nerve damage and the various surgical options are explored.

Trabeculectomy (TM) has been the standard surgical approach since its first description by Cairns [3]. Although it is a successful operation in terms of IOP control [4,5], it has been associated with a considerable number of early and late complications [6] and this has given rise to the development of newer techniques with less complications. The Ex-PRESS glaucoma implant, on the other hand, is made of stainless steel and does not have an internal valve mechanism.

The measurement of the IOP with the Goldmann applanation tonometer (GAT) is the standard clinical practice despite the existence of numerous other tonometers. The optimal area of applanation is based on the Imbert-Fick principle and assumes that the cornea is perfectly elastic, infinitely thin, and dry [7]. As the cornea has none of these features, the accuracy of the measurements with the GAT is limited [7].

Research has shown that the cornea is a more complex structure than a simple elastic surface but also has viscous properties that make the cornea a perplex viscoelastic tissue [8]. The influence of these properties is far higher than the influence of the central cornea thickness and curvature [9]. The Ocular Response Analyzer (ORA; AMETEK Inc. and Reichert Inc., Depew, NY, USA) is a device that can measure both the IOP and the biomechanical properties of the cornea.

The principle of its function relies on the emission of a precisely metered air pulse of 20 ms duration [10]. The ORA has a coupled infrared transmitter, which radiates infrared light on the cornea. This light is reflected by the corneal surface and is detected by the receiver. When the pressure on the cornea by the air jet is such that it applanates the central 3 mm of the corneal surface, then the detected infrared light intensity is maximum and this point corresponds to the inward applanation (P1). The pressure of the air jet continues to increase for a few more milliseconds and then gradually decreases until the cornea becomes flat again due to its elastic properties. At this point, the infrared light intensity is maximum again and the instrument measures the outward applanation pressure (P2). The ORA uses two indices to measure the corneal biomechanical properties: (i) The corneal hysteresis (CH), which is a measure of the viscoelastic properties, and (ii) the corneal resistance factor (CRF), which sums up the effects of the corneal material properties, central corneal thickness and curvature [11]. The CH is calculated as P1−P2 and the CRF is derived from the equation P1−kP2, where k is a constant. When the constant is calculated at $k = 0.68$, then the CRF has its maximum association with the central corneal thickness (CCT) [12]. The ORA offers two different methods of measuring the IOP. The IOP(g) is the average of P1 and P2. The IOP(cc) is calculated from the equation P2-kP1 where k is a constant, which when given the value of 0.43, it is the least dependent on the corneal thickness [12.Within this context, the primary objective of this study was to assess whether the two antiglaucoma procedures (TM and the insertion of the Ex-PRESS mini shunt) affect the biomechanical properties of the cornea differently.

2. Experimental Section

2.1. Setting

This was a prospective, comparative study. Study protocol adhered to the tenets of the Helsinki Declaration and written informed consent was obtained by all participants. The institutional review board of the Democritus University of Thrace approved the protocol (ethical approval code: ES8/Th11/10-10-2013) and study was conducted at the University Hospital of Alexandroupolis (UHA), in Greece between July 2013 and May 2016. Official registration number of the study is NCT04648943.

2.2. Participants

Participants were recruited from the Glaucoma Service of the UHA in a consecutive-if-eligible basis and populated two distinct groups for the purposes of this study: (i) Group 1: Eyes having an Ex-PRESS shunt inserted, and (ii) Group 2: Eyes that underwent TM. Exclusion criteria for both groups included previous ocular trauma, ocular surgery other than phacoemulsification, previous disease of the ocular surface, and congenital glaucoma.

The examination time points for both groups were 1 to 3 weeks preoperatively and 1 month, 6 months, and 12 months postoperatively. All patients had a thorough ophthalmic examination at all time points and the corneal biomechanical properties were measured with the ORA by a trained technician. The ORA measurements were taken before the instillation of the anesthetic drops for the IOP measurement with the GAT. Measurements with a Waveform Score ≤ 3.5 were excluded.

2.3. Surgical Technique-Postoperative Management

All operations were performed by two experienced surgeons (VK, AK) in a consistent way. The surgical technique for the TM was as follows: A conjunctival peritomy was done at the limbus with blunt dissection of the conjunctiva/tenon's capsule. Unipolar cautery was kept to a minimum. A 4 × 4 mm limbus-based flap was formed at roughly half the sclera thickness. Mitomycin C (MMC 0.2 mg/mL for 2–3 min) was applied with the use of a few pieces of a Weck-cell sponge arranged over a wide area under the conjunctiva. The edges of the conjunctiva were grasped with serrated forceps and were wiped with clean Weck-cell sponges. The area of application of MMC was then irrigated with 20 mL of balanced salt solution in order to wash away the MMC. A side port was created with a 20 G knife. Two 10/0 Nylon sutures were preplaced at the corners of the scleral flap. The anterior chamber was entered under the flap with a 45° knife. A corneoscleral block of tissue was excised with a Kelly punch in order to create the internal ostium. A peripheral iridotomy was performed with scissors. More 10/0 Nylon sutures may be placed to the flap according to the surgeon's discretion. The conjunctiva was closed with 2 to 4 10/0 Nylon sutures. Dispersive viscoelastic was injected under the conjunctiva to create a space between the conjunctiva and the sclera for the first postoperative days. A long-acting solution of betamethasone was injected under the conjunctiva behind the filtering bleb and intracameral antibiotic was also used.

There are several models of the implant but in the current study the P50 model was used. It has an internal diameter of 50μm, an external diameter of 0.4 mm, and is 2.46 mm long. The use of this mini shunt has shown to be as effective as the standard TM with fewer side effects [13,14]. The surgical technique for the insertion of the Ex-PRESS mini shunt was the same with the only differences being that the anterior chamber was entered under the flap with a 25 G needle at the anterior part of the blue transition zone (which internally corresponds to the trabeculum). The mini shunt was inserted through the track created by the needle. A peripheral iridotomy was not required.

Topical steroids were prescribed every 2 h tapered gradually according to the surgeon's discretion. Topical antibiotics were prescribed 4 times/day for 1 month. Topical cyclopentolate 1% was given to the trabeculectomy group but not to the Ex-PRESS group as the postoperative inflammation in the latter group is minimal.

The patients were examined in the first postoperative day and at the predetermined time points as mentioned above. At each time point, the surgeon injected dexamethasone with or without 5-fluorouracil and performed needling to the filtering bleb according to his discretion.

2.4. Data Collection

All parameters were measured before surgery and at 1, 6, and 12 months after surgery. The primary outcome measures were the CRF and the CH measured with the use of the ORA, while the secondary outcome measure was the IOP measured with the GAT.

2.5. Statistical Analysis

Medcalc software version 18.2.1 (MedCalc Software bvba, Ostend, Belgium) was used for the statistical analysis. Data distribution was tested with Shapiro–Wilk test and Q-Q plot and parametric and non-parametric tests were applied accordingly. Data are presented as mean ± standard deviation (SD) or error (SE) when the distribution was normal or as median (minimum-maximum) when the distribution was skewed. The power of all statistical tests used was greater than 0.8, suggesting that the size of our sample was sufficient (G*Power 3.1.9.2, University of Dusseldorf, Dusseldorf, Germany). p-values < 0.05 were defined as statistically significant.

3. Results

Thirty patients (30 eyes) were included in the study. Nineteen eyes had an Ex-PRESS shunt inserted (Group 1) and 11 eyes underwent TM (Group 2). Detailed demographic and clinical parameters of each group are presented in Table 1. Non-significant differences were detected with respect to age ($p = 0.18$). No ocular parameter demonstrated significant differences between the two groups preoperatively (p values: 0.2 to 0.43).

Table 1. Demographic characteristics and ocular parameters of the two groups preoperatively.

Demographics and Ocular Parameters	Ex-PRESS	Trabeculectomy	p Value
Sex (M/F)	10/9	6/5	
Age: range (mean)	16–81(62.4)	60–78 (67.2)	0.18
Diagnosis			
• POAG	11	7	
• PXG	8	4	
Pre-op IOP (mean ± SD) (mmHg)	29.4 ± 7.39	33.2 ± 8.61	0.2
Pre-op antiglaucoma agents (mean ± SD)	2.2 ± 0.7	2.3 ± 0.6	
Pre-op CH (mean ± SD)	7.31 ± 1.13	7.82 ± 2.55	0.24
Pre-op CRF (mean ± SD)	10.25 ± 2.76	11.11 ± 1.99	0.43

CH: Corneal hysteresis, CRF: Corneal resistance factor, M: Male, F: Female, IOP: Intraocular pressure, POAG: Primary open angle glaucoma, PXG: Pseudoexfoliation glaucoma, SD: Standard deviation.

In group 1, the data were analyzed with parametric indices using the ANOVA test. The CH was significantly increased at 6 and 12-month time points compared to baseline values (Table 2). CH was also higher at 1 month postoperatively, but this increase did not reach statistical significance. The mean CH was 7.31 preoperatively and increased to 7.92 at 1 month to 8.32 at 6 months and 8.37 at 12 months. On the other hand, CRF was decreased significantly at all time points postoperatively compared to the preoperative values (Table 3). The mean preoperative CRF was 10.6, at 1 month it was 8.07, at 6 months 8.12, and at 12 months 8.35.

Table 2. Corneal hysteresis in group 1 (Ex-press group) at different time points.

CH (Mean)	CH	Mean Difference	SE	p Value [a] (Repeated Measures ANOVA)
Preop: 7.31	Postop—1 month	0.606	0.308	0.394
	—6 months	1.011	0.316	0.0318
	—12 months	1.056	0.313	0.0218

[a]: p value Bonferroni corrected, p values < 0.05 are bold, CH: corneal hysteresis, SE: standard error.

Table 3. Corneal resistance factor in group 1 (Ex-PRESS group) at different time points.

CRF (Mean)	CRF	Mean Difference	SE	p Value [a] (Repeated Measures ANOVA)
Preop: 10.26	Postop—1 month	−2.178	0.540	0.0052
	—6 months	−2.133	0.482	0.0022
	—12 months	−1.9	0.479	0.0060

[a]: p value Bonferroni corrected, p values < 0.05 are bold, CRF: corneal resistance factor.

In group 2, the CH the data were analyzed with non-parametric indices due to the small sample using the Friedman test. The CH was significantly increased at all time points compared to the preoperative values (Table 4). The median preoperative CH was 7.85, at 1 month 8.9, at 6 months 8.8, and at 12 months 8.6. The CRF in the same group was analyzed with the ANOVA test for parametric data. The mean preoperative CRF was 11.11 and it was decreased to 8.21 at the first postoperative month, 8.33 at 6 months, and 8.29 at 1 year. The decrease of the CRF was significant at all time points compared to the preoperative values (Table 5).

Table 4. Corneal hysteresis in group 2 at different time points.

CH	Median	Minimum–Maximum	CH Preop—Time Points	p Value [a] (Friedman Test)
preop	7.85	3.9–13.9	Preop	
1 month	8.9	6.2–14.7	—1 month	p value < 0.05
6 months	8.8	6.4–14	—6 months	
12 months	8.6	6.6–14.8	—12 months	

[a]: Conover post—hoc test, CH: corneal hysteresis.

Table 5. Corneal resistance factor in group 2 at different time points.

CRF (Mean)	CRF	Mean Difference	SE	p Value [a] (Repeated Measures ANOVA)
Preop: 11.11	Preop—1 month	2.9	0.548	0.0015
	—6 months	2.783	0.438	0.0003
	—12 months	2.825	0.422	0.0002

[a]: p value Bonferroni corrected, p values < 0.05 are highlighted, CRF: corneal resistance factor, SE: standard error.

We performed a regression analysis to check for any correlation of the CH and CRF change taking into account the IOP change. With GAT-IOP as a covariate, we found that the CH and CRF change (before and after surgery) in both groups was not significant at all time points (all $p < 0.05$).

We also carried out multivariate analysis using a linear regression model, with a stepwise backward elimination procedure including changes in IOP, CH, CRF, and patients' age in order to find any correlation between these variables. Multivariate analysis did not reveal any correlation between changes in biomechanical properties (CH, CRF) and patients' age and/or IOP changes.

Finally, we compared the difference (preoperative values to postoperative values at all time points) of the CH between the two groups (Welch test) and we did not detect any significant differences between the two surgical techniques (Table 6). When the CRF changes (preoperative values to postoperative values at all time points) were compared between the two groups (using the t-test), they were not found to be significant (Table 7).

Table 6. Difference of the corneal hysteresis (CH) values (preoperative values to postoperative values at all time points) for the two groups.

CH (Preop-postop Time Points)	1 Month Mean ± SD	p Value (Welch Test)	6 Months Mean ± SD	p Value (Welch Test)	12 Months Mean ± SD	p Value (Welch Test)
Ex-PRESS group	0.75 ± 2.23	0.44	1.59 ± 2.82	0.56	1.64 ± 2.82	0.47
Trab group	1.22 ± 1.08		1.15 ± 1.11		1.1 ± 1.06	

CH: Corneal hysteresis, SD: Standard deviation.

Table 7. Difference of the corneal resistance factor (CRF) values (preoperative values to postoperative values at all time points) for the two groups.

CRF (Preop-Postop Time Points)	1 Month Mean ± SD	p Value (Unpaired t-Test)	6 Months Mean ± SD	p Value (Unpaired t-Test)	12 Months Mean ± SD	p Value (Unpaired t-Test)
Ex-PRESS group	−1.67 ± 2.7	0.23	−2.13 ± 2.04	0.62	−1.9 ± 2.03	0.27
Trab group	−2.9 ± 1.89		−1.7 ± 2.7		−2.81 ± 1.47	

CRF: Corneal resistance factor, SD: Standard deviation.

The IOP was significantly reduced at all postoperative time points with both procedures. The difference in the hypotensive effect between the 2 procedures was similar for both procedures (Table 8).

Table 8. Mean intraocular pressure (IOP) before and after surgery at the predetermined time points for the two groups.

Mean IOP	Trabeculectomy (Mean ± SD)		ExPRESS (Mean ± SD)		p Value (Unpaired t-Test)
Preop	33.2 ± 8.61		29.4 ± 7.39		0.2
—1 month	10.4 ± 4.86		12.9 ± 4.57		0.16
—6 months	13.6 ± 4.1	p value < 0.05	15.9 ± 3.23	p value < 0.05	0.10
—12 months	15.9 ± 3.07		16.1 ± 3.77		0.87

IOP: Intraocular pressure, SD: Standard deviation.

Three patients in group 2 needed two antiglaucoma agents to achieve adequate hypotensive effect and one patient in group 1 needed one drop.

Three eyes in the TM group had hypotension (<6 mmHg) in the early postoperative period but only one of them was taken back to operating theatre and more sutures were placed to the scleral flap. Two patients in the Ex-PRESS group had hypotension but were managed conservatively.

4. Discussion

In this study, we investigated the effect of the two antiglaucoma procedures on the corneal biomechanical properties. We found that both indices of the corneal biomechanical properties (CH and CRF) changed significantly in the postoperative period and these changes were similar in both groups. None of the indices returned to the preoperative values 1 year after surgery.

Corneal hysteresis is an indicator of the viscous properties of the cornea, which are due to the presence of glycosaminoglycans, the proteoglycans, and the extracellular matrix [15]. Its value in non-diseased eyes in adult population is around 10.2 mmHg [16]. Regarding its significance in glaucoma, numerous studies agree that CH is lower in eyes with POAG, ocular hypertension, and normal tension glaucoma [17]. Corneal hysteresis was related to glaucomatous field damage progression [18] as well as functional deterioration in the form of reduction of the retinal nerve fiber thickness [19]. In addition to the above, the biomechanical properties of the surface of the eye may reflect similar properties of the lamina cribrosa (LC) of the optic nerve. Lower CH values mean that the cornea (or other tissues like LC) cannot absorb the energy that is exercised on them efficiently and deform at a great extent. On the other hand, tissues with high CH can absorb energy efficiently and do not deform as much. Eyes with lower CH are more prone to glaucomatous damage of the optic nerve as the connective tissue around it deforms significantly (compared to eyes with high CH) as a result of the effect of the IOP and this can lead to damage of optic nerve fibers that run through the LC [20].

Research bears conflicting results regarding the relationship of baseline CH and GAT-IOP. Touboul et al. [21] compared the correlation between GAT-IOP and CH in five groups (normal, glaucoma, keratocus, laser in situ keratomileusis, photorefractive keratectomy) and found a strong correlation only in the glaucoma group. Kaushik at al. [22] analyzed the correlation of CH and GAT-IOP in a cohort comprised of normal subjects, glaucoma suspects, ocular hypertensives, primary angle closure disease, POAG, and normal tension glaucoma patients and found a strong correlation between the two variables. Regarding to the key issue of which device clinicians should use to measure the IOP, Pillunat et al. [23] argue that GAT underestimates the IOP by 3–4 mmHg after trabeculectomy and that IOPcc is a more reliable index of the real IOP. On the other hand, Kaushik et al. [22] believe that the Goldmann tonometer should be used in routine practice. Given the fact the ORA is not widely available in many ophthalmological settings and for an accurate measurement of the IOP and the corneal biomechanical indices to be obtained, a reliable measurement must be taken with the ORA [24], it seems that the Goldmann tonometer is an accurate and at the same time easily accessible instrument. The authors of this study believe that in some cases where the clinical picture of a patient demands an in-depth measurement and evaluation of multiple variables, then in such a case, it would be advisable to use the ORA as well.

The importance of these properties lies in the fact that they affect the measurements of the IOP to a greater effect than the central corneal thickness [25]. As the IOP reduction is the main target of the antiglaucoma operations, it is of paramount significance that the clinician can estimate as accurately as possible the true IOP. The effect of phacoemulsification on the corneal biomechanical properties has been measured in other studies. de Freitas et al. [26] found that the CH temporarily decreases in the immediate postoperative period but returns to the preoperative values later. CRF on the other hand decreased significantly but its values did not return to the preoperative levels at the end of the study period. Zhang et al. [27] also found that CH returned to the preoperative values after a decrease for a short period of time. They did not observe, however, any significant changes of the CRF.

Several other investigators looked at the effect of the antiglaucoma surgeries on the cornea. Sun et al. [28] found that the CH increases in eyes with chronic primary angle closure glaucoma after TM and this tendency remains constant four weeks after surgery. In another study, the influence of TM on the CH and CRF were investigated by Pillunat et al. [23]. Neither of the indices changed significantly postoperatively although there was a trend for reduction of both indices. Interestingly, both IOP measurements given by the ORA (IOPcc and IOPg) were significantly higher than Goldmann tonometry.

However, in TM, surgeons do not insert a drainage device. In this study, we included a group that had an Ex-PRESS implant inserted under a scleral flap in order to achieve IOP reduction. We found one study in which the effects on the cornea of a drainage device were measured. Pakravan et al. [29] compared the effects of TM, combined phacoemulsification-TM (PT), Ahmed drainage device, and phacoemulsification on the cornea. They reported that CH increased in all groups three months postoperatively, while CRF decreased. They speculated that the reasons for the increase of the CH are the reduction of the IOP and the discontinuation of the topical antiglaucoma medication. The latter have been found to cause an increase of the CH [30,31], which does not explain the higher CH values after a successful antiglaucoma procedure.

In order to investigate whether the increase of the biomechanical markers was due to the decrease of the IOP, we performed a regression analysis taking into account the IOP change. According to our data, the change of both indices (before and after surgery) was not correlated to the IOP change (before and after surgery). Multivariate analysis taking into account the GAT-IOP and age did not show any correlation with the biomechanical properties. According to our results, it seems that the glaucoma procedures affect the integrity of the cornea permanently. This is to be expected as less invasive procedures such as uneventful phacoemulsification does alter the corneal structure even if this is only temporary [25]. We would not expect to witness these structural changes at the level of lacrimal cribrosa as the consequences of the glaucoma surgery have local effects and not global.

Our results agree with the results of previous studies in terms of an increase of the CH after antiglaucoma surgery. However, we found that the CRF decreased postoperatively in both groups and this trend remained the same for the entire study period. A similar effect was noted by Pillunat et al. [31] after selective laser trabeculoplasty. CH and CRF measure different properties of the cornea and they are influenced by different factors. CH represents the viscous properties and the CRF the elastic. The reason for the decrement of the CRF values can be the fact that the cornea becomes less elastic after surgery due to effect of the remodeling of the ocular tissues as a response to ocular trauma.

It has been shown that the CH can increase or decrease as the cornea becomes stiffer (old age, cross linking) [32,33]. The role of the CH as an indicator of the corneal stiffness has been debated. There are other factors that influence corneal stiffness (other than viscosity) such as elasticity, hydration, thickness, and extracellular material. However, the increase of the CH after reduction of the IOP (irrespective of its cause) has been shown in many studies [27–32]. The alterations of the CRF in our study seem to represent the influence of the surgery and/or the presence of a foreign body (Ex-PRESS mini-shunt) in the vicinity of the cornea.

Our study has several limitations. The small sample size of the two groups is a limiting factor in making safe deductions about the effect of the TM and the Ex-PRESS device on the cornea. We also have not taken into account the IOP as a covariate in the statistical analysis of the CH and CRF. On the other hand, we followed up our patients for a year, which is longer than the follow-up period in similar studies.

5. Conclusions

In summary, both surgical techniques have shown to cause an increase of the CH to the same extent postoperatively and a decrease of the CRF. Clinicians should bear in mind these biomechanical changes after an antiglaucoma procedure and adapt their postoperative evaluation and plan accordingly.

Author Contributions: Conceptualization, A.K.; methodology, A.K.; software, E.-K.P. and H.S.; validation, G.L.; formal analysis G.D.P.; investigation, H.S. and A.M.; resources: G.D.P.; data curation, G.D.P. and A.K.; writing—original draft preparation, A.K.; writing—review and editing, G.L. and E.-K.P.; visualization, A.M. and E.-K.P.; supervision, G.L.; project administration, A.K.; funding acquisition, n/a. All authors have read and agreed to the published version of the manuscript.

Funding: This research received no external funding.

Institutional Review Board Statement: The institutional review board of the Democritus University of Thrace unanimously decides to approve the elaboration of the study the "The Effect of Antiglaucoma Procedures (Trabeculectomy vs. Ex-PRESS Glaucoma Drainage Implant) on the Corneal Biomechanical Properties and on the macular architecture" in the context of Aristeidis Konstantinidis's PhD thesis. The study will be conducted in the University Eye Clinic of the University Hospital of Alexandroupolis, Greece. (ethical approval code: ES8/Th11/10-10-2019).

Informed Consent Statement: Informed consent was obtained from all subjects involved in the study.

Data Availability Statement: Authors are willing to share the individual deidentified participant data including written consent forms and study information leaflets for at least one year following the publication of our manuscript, acceptable in print form. Please note that all relevant data is in Greek language.

Conflicts of Interest: The authors declare no conflict of interest.

References

1. Resnikoff, S.; Pascolini, D.; Etya'ale, D.; Kocur, I.; Pararajasegaram, R.; Pokharel, G.P.; Mariotti, S.P. Global data on visual impairment in the year 2002. *Bull World Health Organ.* **2004**, *82*, 844–851.
2. Leske, M.C.; Connell, A.M.; Wu, S.Y.; Hyman, L.G.; Schachat, A.P. Risk factors for open-angle glaucoma. The Barbados Eye Study. *Arch. Ophthalmol.* **1995**, *113*, 918–924. [CrossRef]
3. Cairns, J.E. Trabeculectomy. Preliminary report of a new method. *Am. J. Ophthalmol.* **1968**, *66*, 673–679. [CrossRef]
4. Jampel, H.D.; Solus, J.F.; Tracey, P.A.; Gilbert, D.L.; Loyd, T.L.; Jefferys J.L.; Quigley, H.A. Outcomes and bleb-related complications of trabeculectomy. *Ophthalmology* **2012**, *119*, 712–722. [CrossRef]
5. Fontana, H.; Nouri-Mahdavi, K.; Lumba, J.; Ralli, M.; Caprioli, J. Trabeculectomy with mitomycin C: Outcomes and risk factors for failure in phakic open-angle glaucoma. *Ophthalmology* **2006**, *113*, 930–936. [CrossRef]
6. Edmunds, B.; Thompson, J.R.; Salmon, J.F.; Wormald, R.P. The National Survey of Trabeculectomy. III. Early and late complications. *Eye* **2002**, *16*, 297–303. [CrossRef] [PubMed]
7. Kohlhaas, M.; Boehm, A.G.; Spoerl, E.; Pürsten, A.; Grein, H.J.; Pillunat, L.E. Effect of central corneal thickness, corneal curvature, and axial length on applanation tonometry. *Arch. Ophthalmol.* **2006**, *124*, 471–476. [CrossRef]
8. Soergel, F.; Jean, B.; Seiler, T.; Bende, T.; Mücke, S.; Pechhold, W.; Fels, L. Dynamic mechanical spectroscopy of the cornea for measurement of its viscoelastic properties in vitro. *Ger. J. Ophthalmol.* **1995**, *4*, 151–156.
9. Liu, J.; Roberts, C.J. Influence of corneal biomechanical properties on intraocular pressure measurement: Quantitative analysis. *J. Cataract. Refract. Surg.* **2005**, *31*, 146–155. [CrossRef] [PubMed]
10. Luce, D.A. Determining in vivo biomechanical properties of the cornea with an ocular response analyzer. *J. Cataract. Refract. Surg.* **2005**, *31*, 156–162. [CrossRef]

11. Medeiros, F.A.; Weinreb, R.N. Evaluation of the influence of corneal biomechanical properties on intraocular pressure measurements using the ocular response analyzer. *J. Glaucoma* **2006**, *15*, 364–370. [CrossRef]
12. Kotecha, A.; Elsheikh, A.; Roberts, C.R.; Zhu, H.; Garway-Heath, D.F. Corneal thickness- and age-related biomechanical properties of the cornea measured with the ocular response analyzer. *Investig. Ophthalmol. Vis. Sci.* **2006**, *47*, 5337–5347. [CrossRef]
13. Dahan, E.; Ben Simon, G.J.; Lafuma, A. Comparison of trabeculectomy and Ex-PRESS implantation in fellow eyes of the same patient: A prospective, randomised study. *Eye* **2012**, *26*, 703–710. [CrossRef]
14. Marzette, L.; Herndon, L.W. Comparison of the Ex-PRESS™ mini glaucoma shunt with standard trabeculectomy in the surgical treatment of glaucoma. *Ophthalmic. Surg. Lasers Imaging* **2011**, *42*, 453–459. [CrossRef]
15. Terai, N.; Raiskup, F.; Haustein, M.; Pillunat, L.E.; Spoerl, E. Identification of biomechanical properties of the cornea: The ocular response analyzer. *Curr. Eye Res.* **2012**, *37*, 553–562. [CrossRef]
16. Carbonaro, F.; Andrew, T.; Mackey, D.A.; Spector, T.D.; Hammond, C.J. The heritability of corneal hysteresis and ocular pulse amplitude: A twin study. *Ophthalmology* **2008**, *115*, 1545–1549. [CrossRef]
17. Liang, L.; Zhang, R.; He, L.-Y. Corneal hysteresis and glaucoma. *Int. Ophthalmol.* **2019**, *39*, 1909–1916. [CrossRef]
18. Congdon, N.G.; Broman, A.T.; Bandeen-Roche, K.; Grover, D.; Quigley, H.A. Central corneal thickness and corneal hysteresis associated with glaucoma damage. *Am. J. Ophthalmol.* **2006**, *141*, 868–875. [CrossRef]
19. Zhang, C.; Tatham, A.J.; Abe, R.Y.; Diniz-Filho, A.; Zangwill, L.M.; Weinreb, R.N.; Medeiros, F.A. Corneal hysteresis and progressive retinal nerve fiber layer loss in glaucoma. *Am. J. Ophthalmol.* **2016**, *166*, 29–36. [CrossRef]
20. Zimprich, L.; Diedrich, J.; Bleeker, A.; Schweitzer, J.A. Corneal Hysteresis as a Biomarker of Glaucoma: Current Insights. *Clin. Ophthalmol.* **2020**, *14*, 2255–2264. [CrossRef]
21. Touboul, D.; Roberts, C.; Kérautret, J.; Garra, C.; Maurice-Tison, S.; Saubusse, E.; Colin, J. Correlations between corneal hysteresis, intraocular pressure, and corneal central pachymetry. *J. Cataract Refract. Surg.* **2015**, *30*, 335–339. [CrossRef]
22. Kaushik, S.; Pandav, S.S.; Banger, A.; Aggarwal, K.; Gupta, A. Relationship between corneal biomechanical properties, central corneal thickness, and intraocular pressure across the spectrum of glaucoma. *Am. J. Ophthalmol.* **2012**, *153*, 840–849. [CrossRef]
23. Pillunat, K.R.; Spoerl, E.; Terai, N.; Pillunat, L.E. Corneal Biomechanical Changes After Trabeculectomy and the Impact on Intraocular Pressure Measurement. *J. Glaucoma* **2017**, *26*, 278–282. [CrossRef] [PubMed]
24. Ayala, M.; Chen, E. Measuring corneal hysteresis: Threshold estimation of the waveform score from the Ocular Response Analyzer. *Graefes Arch. Clin. Exp. Ophthalmol.* **2012**, *250*, 1803–1806. [CrossRef]
25. de Freitas Valbon, B.; Ventura, M.P.; da Silva, R.S.; Canedo, A.L.; Velarde, G.C.; Ambrósio, R., Jr. Central corneal thickness and biomechanical changes after clear corneal phacoemulsification. *J. Refract. Surg.* **2012**, *28*, 215–219. [CrossRef]
26. Zhang, Z.; Yu, H.; Dong, H.; Wang, L.; Jia, Y.D.; Zhang, S.H. Corneal biomechanical properties changes after coaxial 2.2-mm microincision and standard 3.0-mm phacoemulsification. *Int. J. Ophthalmol.* **2016**, *9*, 230–234. [CrossRef]
27. Sun, L.; Shen, M.; Wang, J.; Fang, A.; Xu, A.; Fang, H.; Lu, F. Recovery of corneal hysteresis after reduction of intraocular pressure in chronic primary angle-closure glaucoma. *Am. J. Ophthalmol.* **2009**, *147*, 1061–1066. [CrossRef]
28. Pakravan, M.; Afroozifar, M.; Yazdani, S. Corneal Biomechanical Changes Following Trabeculectomy, Phaco-trabeculectomy, Ahmed Glaucoma Valve Implantation and Phacoemulsification. *J. Ophthalmic. Vis. Res.* **2014**, *9*, 7–13.
29. Bolívar, G.; Sánchez-Barahona, C.; Teus, M.; Castejón, M.A.; Paz-Moreno-Arrones, J.; Gutiérrez-Ortiz, C.; Mikropoulos, D.G. Effect of topical prostaglandin analogues on corneal hysteresis. *Acta Ophthalmol.* **2015**, *93*, e495–e498. [CrossRef]
30. Tsikripis, P.; Papaconstantinou, D.; Koutsandrea, C.; Apostolopoulos, M.; Georgalas, I. The effect of prostaglandin analogs on the biomechanical properties and central thickness of the cornea of patients with open-angle glaucoma: A 3-year study on 108 eyes. *Drug Des. Devel. Ther.* **2013**, *7*, 1149–1156. [CrossRef] [PubMed]
31. Pillunat, K.R.; Spoerl, E.; Terai, N.; Pillunat, L.E. Effect of selective laser trabeculoplasty on corneal biomechanics. *Acta. Ophthalmol.* **2016**, *94*, e501–e504. [CrossRef]
32. Sahin, A.; Bayer, A. Corneal hysteresis changes in diabetic eyes. *J. Cataract. Refract. Surg.* **2010**, *36*, 361–362. [CrossRef]
33. Sharifipour, F.; Panahi-Bazaz, M.; Bidar, R.; Idani, A.; Cheraghian, B. Age-related variations in corneal biomechanical properties. *J. Curr. Ophthalmol.* **2016**, *28*, 117–122. [CrossRef]

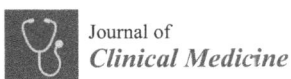

Article

Phacotrabeculectomy versus Phaco with Implantation of the Ex-PRESS Device: Surgical and Refractive Outcomes—A Randomized Controlled Trial

Joanna Konopińska [1,*], Anna Byszewska [2], Emil Saeed [1], Zofia Mariak [1] and Marek Rękas [2]

1. Department of Ophthalmology, Medical University of Białystok, M. Sklodowska-Curie 24A STR, 15-276 Białystok, Poland; emilsaeed1986@gmail.com (E.S.); mariakzo@umb.edu.pl (Z.M.)
2. Department of Ophthalmology, Military Institute of Medicine, Szaserów 128 STR, 04-141 Warszawa, Poland; ania.byszewska@gmail.com (A.B.); rekasp.@gmail.com (M.R.)
* Correspondence: joannakonopinska@o2.pl; Tel.: +48-857468372

Abstract: The aim of this study was to compare surgical and refractive outcomes between phacotrabeculectomy (P-Trab) and phaco with Ex-PRESS (P-Ex-PRESS) for glaucoma at a 6-month follow-up. This prospective randomized controlled trial included 81 eyes; 43 eyes (53%) and 38 eyes (47%) were assigned to the P-Ex-PRESS and P-Trab groups, respectively. Refraction, intraocular pressure (IOP), and best-corrected visual acuity were measured. Refractive change was analyzed using the cylinder's magnitude, and polar analysis assessed the change in the trend of astigmatism [with-the-rule, against-the-rule (ATR), oblique (OBL)], evaluating mean astigmatism in centroid form. All patients showed a statistically significant postoperative decrease in IOP ($P < 0.05$). There were no differences between the groups in terms of postoperative IOP and visual outcomes or in astigmatism preoperatively or postoperatively ($P = 0.61$, $P = 0.74$). In both groups, the mean preoperative and postoperative astigmatism were ATR and OBL, respectively. Preoperative and postoperative centroids in the P-Ex-PRESS group were 0.44 ± 1.32 D at 177° and 0.35 ± 1 D at 8°, respectively, ($P = 0.5$) and in the P-Trab group were 0.16 ± 1.5 D at 141° and 0.39 ± 1.38 D at 29°, respectively ($P = 0.38$). Both P-Ex-PRESS and P-Trab showed comparable antihypertensive efficacy in treating open-angle glaucoma over 6 months. Preoperative and postoperative astigmatism did not differ between groups. The groups showed comparable results for final visual acuity.

Keywords: astigmatism; glaucoma; intraocular pressure; phacotrabeculectomy; Ex-PRESS device

Citation: Konopińska, J.; Byszewska, A.; Saeed, E.; Mariak, Z.; Rękas, M. Phacotrabeculectomy versus Phaco with Implantation of the Ex-PRESS Device: Surgical and Refractive Outcomes—A Randomized Controlled Trial. *J. Clin. Med.* **2021**, *10*, 424. https://doi.org/10.3390/jcm10030424

Academic Editor: Georgios Labiris
Received: 5 December 2020
Accepted: 19 January 2021
Published: 22 January 2021

Publisher's Note: MDPI stays neutral with regard to jurisdictional claims in published maps and institutional affiliations.

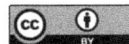

Copyright: © 2021 by the authors. Licensee MDPI, Basel, Switzerland. This article is an open access article distributed under the terms and conditions of the Creative Commons Attribution (CC BY) license (https://creativecommons.org/licenses/by/4.0/).

1. Introduction

Trabeculectomy and implantation of the Ex-PRESS mini device (Alcon Laboratories, Fort Worth, TX, USA) are anti-glaucoma procedures that improve subconjunctival outflow [1]. Although trabeculectomy remains the "gold standard" for anti-glaucoma surgery, implantation of the less-invasive Ex-PRESS mini seton is also effective [2]. Both procedures establish a new, alternative outflow route within the trabecular meshwork and evacuation of the aqueous humor via artificial filtering fistulae. They can be used as a standalone procedure or combined with phacoemulsification when patients have both glaucoma and cataract. A simultaneous approach can reduce the anesthesia and surgery time, with less recovery time and reduced overall cost of care to the patient and the health system [3]. Penetrating glaucoma procedures require extended ocular tissue interference, such as conjunctival preparation, scleral cutting, and suture application. However, they provide high hypotensive efficacy, and are reasonable treatments for moderate to advanced glaucoma, eliminating the chronic need for intraocular pressure (IOP)-lowering eye drops. Patients undergoing glaucoma surgery often have a brief period of reduced visual acuity in the early postoperative period, which can persist on a long term basis in some cases [4]. This could be due to surgically induced astigmatism (SIA) after penetrating glaucoma procedures such as trabeculectomy [5–7]. The degree of astigmatism may be influenced by the surgical technique (i.e., scleral flap size), the sutures used for conjunctival closure (mattress vs. knotted), suture tightness, use of cauterization, the cauterization technique (dry vs. wet), the duration of surgery, the trabeculectomy tool used (punch vs. knife), and use of anti-metabolites (dose and time) [7]. Moreover, IOP fluctuations in the postoperative period, caused by the pressure of the upper eyelid on the filtering bleb, may also induce astigmatism [7,8]. With-the-rule (WTR) astigmatism after phacotrabeculectomy (P-Trab) can worsen postoperative visual acuity [9,10]. Implantation of Ex-PRESS device combined with phaco (P-Ex-PRESS) differs in that it does not require cutting a fragment of the sclera, limbus, or iris or the use of a punch. Some authors report that this may reduce wound gape and "sinking" due to tissue removal [3]. Therefore, it remains unclear whether P-Ex-PRESS surgery generates less astigmatism than P-Trab surgery. Several studies have assessed SIA after trabeculectomy, non-penetrating surgery, or minimally invasive glaucoma surgery, with most studies obtaining data through a retrospective chart review without a control group. There is no clear data on refractive outcomes of Ex-PRESS device surgery, and no study has evaluated the refractive outcomes of combined Ex-PRESS implants and cataract surgery versus P-Trab in a prospective design Our study aimed to compare the amount of SIA and refractive change in P-Trab versus P-Ex-PRESS surgery to evaluate the relative surgical success of these procedures in a randomized, controlled trial with a 6-month follow-up. This research contributes much-needed data on the efficacy and safety profile of the Ex-PRESS device in comparison with trabeculectomy.

2. Materials and Methods

2.1. Patients

This study adheres to the tenets of the Declaration of Helsinki and the Principles of Good Clinical Practice developed by the European Union. The study protocol was approved by the Bioethics Committee at the Medical University in Białystok under the number R-I-002/443/2014 and registered on clinicaltrials.gov (registration number: NCT04335825). Written informed consent to participate for at least 6 months was obtained from all patients after an explanation of the nature of the procedure and surgical alternatives. The study protocol was similar to that documented in our previous work [11].

We recruited consecutive patients who were referred to the ophthalmology clinic of our hospital and qualified for combined surgery. Glaucoma with coexisting cataract graded NC1 or NC2 by the Lens Opacities Classification System III scale was the surgical indication. Patients with primary open-angle glaucoma, pseudoexfoliation glaucoma, and pigmentary glaucoma, where target IOP was not achieved, despite maximally-tolerated topical and systemic medication and well-documented visual field defect progression, were eligible for treatment. A patient qualified for surgery if any of the following additional inclusion criteria was present: significant diurnal variations in IOP, poor patient compliance, or allergy to topical anti-glaucoma drugs with progressive visual field loss. The exclusion criteria were as follows: lack of consent for study participation, history of eye surgery or laser procedures within the eye, closed or narrow-angle glaucoma, diabetes, advanced macular degeneration, and active inflammatory disease.

The randomized prospective study included 81 eyes of 81 patients. A computer-generated randomization list was created, with allocation concealment. Randomization was performed using sealed envelopes, opened on the day of surgery, to determine the randomization group. The eyes were individually randomized in a 1:1 ratio to either phacoemulsification with simultaneous Ex-PRESS mini glaucoma shunt implantation (43 eyes (53%)) or P-Trab (38 eyes (47%)).

2.2. Preoperative Examination

Detailed data on patient demographics (age, sex), previous treatments, and surgical procedures were collected at the time of qualification. Before surgical treatment, all patients underwent a basic examination, which included determination of IOP, uncorrected distance visual acuity, best-corrected visual acuity (BCVA), and refractive findings (refractive error: sphere and cylinder with axis), axial length, and biomicroscopic examination of the anterior and posterior eye segments, with a detailed assessment of the retina and optic nerve disc. The BCVA was examined with the Snellen notification and expressed as logMAR units. A Snellen BCVA of 1.0 (100% or 20/20) equals a logMAR of 0.

The intraocular lens (IOL) power was calculated with the IOL Master 700 (Carl Zeiss Meditec, AG, Jena, Germany). All patients were implanted with the same type of IOL. Gonioscopy was performed along with the field of vision test (Humphrey Field Analyzer, program SITA standard 24-2, Carl Zeiss-Humphrey Systems, Dublin, CA, USA). The IOP was measured during preoperative examination using a slit-lamp–mounted Goldmann applanation tonometer in accordance with the Advanced Glaucoma Intervention Study. The reading in mm Hg was rounded to the closest integer. Each measurement was repeated twice, and if the difference between the two readings was ≥ 3 mm Hg, a third measurement was taken. The mean of two or three measurements was used to determine the IOP.

2.3. Surgical Technique

All surgical procedures were performed under retrobulbar anesthesia (2% xylocaine and 0.5% bupivacaine) by the same experienced surgeon (JK) for the duration of the study. In both procedures, the fornix-base conjunctiva was dissected, and the sclera was exposed. A limbus-based, square-shaped (4 mm × 4 mm) scleral flap was dissected using the technique described by Traverso et al. [1]. A clear corneal incision of 2.25 mm was made temporally with the phaco-chop technique for phacoemulsification using the Megatron S4 HPS (Geuder, Heidelberg, Germany), and an IOL was implanted into the capsular bag. The same type of IOLs (Akreos Adapt, Bausch & Lomb, Rochester, NY, USA) were implanted for all surgeries. In the P-Ex-PRESS group, a mini glaucoma shunt was implanted at the one o'clock position, using a technique described previously [12]. In the P-Trab group, iridectomy was made at the same position. The scleral flap was closed with 10/0 nylon sutures (four knotted sutures) and the conjunctival closure was achieved with absorbable sutures. During trabeculectomy and Ex-PRESS mini glaucoma shunt implantation, 5-fluorouracil (5-FU; 50 mg/mL) was used on a standard basis and applied to the scleral wound bed for 3.5 min to avoid contact with the conjunctival incision area [9]

2.4. Postoperative Protocol

During the follow-up visits, the IOP and BCVA were measured, as mentioned above, by the same unmasked resident doctor. Detailed biomicroscopic evaluation of the anterior chamber and fundus of the eye was performed. During the postoperative assessment, both complications and the number of IOP-lowering medications administered were documented. Additional procedures were performed when insufficient filtration was noted as an elevated IOP (≥ 16 mm Hg) or an underdeveloped or completely flat filtering bleb [9]. Inadequate filtration was diagnosed during the first 2 weeks after surgery when healing did not yet restrict subconjunctival outflow and a progressive increase in the IOP >16 mm Hg was observed [9]. Patients were examined for the presence and proper functioning of the filtering bleb and the development of subconjunctival fibrosis (observed as engorged and tortuous blood vessels above the scleral flap). Needling was performed based on a diagnosis of fibrosis (based on the above clinical signs), insufficient subconjunctival outflow, increase in IOP, or flattening of the bleb, by the same examiner throughout the whole follow-up. If fibrosis occurred, 5-FU subconjunctival injections were administered (5 mg in 0.2 mL), combined with needling when appropriate, for 5 consecutive days or until fibrosis disappeared and the IOP stabilized, provided that no anti-metabolite-related adverse effects were encountered [10]. Needling was performed when a flat, dysfunctional filtering bleb was observed. Suture lysis was performed within the first 2 weeks after surgery when poor filtration through the bleb was observed (due to overly tight suturing of the scleral flap). Needling and suture lysis were not considered as failures. An IOP ≤ 6 mm Hg was defined as ocular hypotony.

The success rate was defined as either complete or qualified. Complete surgical success was defined as IOP ≤18 mm Hg without anti-glaucoma medications, whereas qualified success was defined as IOP ≤18 mm Hg with a maximum of two anti-glaucoma medications (determined by the number of active ingredients). In the case of IOP >18 mm Hg with or without anti-glaucoma medications or when the eye required further surgical intervention, surgery was considered a failure. No anti-glaucoma medications were allowed on the day of the operation. When surgery did not achieve the expected results, medications were re-administered as recommended by the European Glaucoma Society rules.

Control examinations were performed both before treatment and on the first and seventh postoperative days, as well as at postoperative days 30, 90, and 180. Postoperatively, all eyes were treated with topical postoperative steroids (Loteprednol, one drop three times daily for 4 weeks), and tapered to twice daily after 1 week. Antibiotic (Moxifloksacin) was administered as a single drop three times daily for 2 weeks and nonsteroidal anti-inflammatory drugs as one drop three times daily for 4 weeks.

2.5. Refractive Data Evaluation

Autorefractometry data from before and 180 days after surgery were included in the analysis. Refractive and vector analyses were performed. Refractive analysis, a simple arithmetic calculation of the mean of the cylinder without considering its axis, was performed to compare with the numerical results available in the literature. This difference in the mean value of the cylinder allows for reporting the mean change in the magnitude of astigmatism. All calculations were performed using the plus form of the cylinder.

The vector analysis is a calculation of the cylinder change considering its axis. The preoperative and postoperative refractive measurements (cylinder with its axis) were evaluated by vector analysis, according to the method proposed by Holladay et al. [13]. Data were converted from standard polar values (cylinder and axis) to Cartesian values (points with x, y coordinates) to evaluate trends in astigmatism (against-the-rule [ATR], WTR, or oblique) and to define mean astigmatism in the centroid form.

For conversion from polar to Cartesian values, the following mathematical formulae were applied:

$$x = cyl \times \cos(2 \times axis)$$

$$y = cyl \times \sin(2 \times axis).$$

Cartesian coordinates were converted to standard polar values using the below formulae:

$$cyl = \sqrt{(x^2 + y^2)}$$
$$angle = \tfrac{1}{2} \times [\tan^{-1}(y/x)]$$

if $x > 0$ and $y > 0$	→	axis = angle
if $x < 0$	→	axis = angle + 90°
if $x > 0$ and $y < 0$	→	axis = angle + 180°
if $x = 0$ and $y < 0$	→	axis = 135°
if $x = 0$ and $y > 0$	→	axis = 45°
if $x = 0$ and $y = 0$	→	axis = 0°
if $y = 0$ and $x < 0$	→	axis = 90°
if $y = 0$ and $x > 0$	→	axis = 0°.

This calculation was performed for each individual to obtain the surgically induced refractive change. The mean of all x and y values were calculated to allow calculation of the aggregate refractive change of the analyzed groups. Data were displayed as double-angle plots because the angles were doubled owing to the return of the astigmatism vector to the same value when traversing 180°.

The major and minor axes of the centroid of the ellipse were determined by calculating the standard deviations of the x and y coordinates. The astigmatism trend was evaluated based on the shape factor and the centroid axis.

The aggregate data considered the mean value of astigmatism (mean magnitude of the cylinder), which does not include the axis analysis or centroid calculation.

The centroid was used to define the direction of astigmatism (WTR, against-the-rule, or oblique).

The double-angle plots were prepared using the double-angle-plot-tool for astigmatism available on the American Society of Cataract and Refractive Surgery website. Data on astigmatism values were depicted in cumulative data plots at 0.5-D intervals.

2.6. Statistical Evaluation

In both groups, quantitative data are expressed as arithmetic means, standard deviations, and medians. Qualitative characteristics are expressed as numbers and percentages. Data were tested for normality using the Shapiro–Wilk test. Between-group comparisons were made using Student's t-test or Mann-Whitney U test. The x^2 test of independence for two variables was used to compare quantitative characteristics. Values of $P < 0.05$ were considered to indicate statistical significance. Analyses were conducted using SPSS version 24.0 (IBM, Armonk, NY, USA).

3. Results

A total of 43 and 38 patients underwent P-Ex-PRESS and P-Trab procedures, respectively. The demographic data are summarized in Table 1.

Table 1. Patient demographic data.

Group.	P-ExPress	P-Trab	P *
Follow-up (months)	6.7 ± 0.4	6.9 ± 0.5	0.249
Number	43	38	-
Age (years)	72.1 ± 4.62	67.2 ± 9.28	0.374
Sex (female/male)	26/17	28/10	0.579
Eye (right/left)	23/20	17/21	0.658
Glaucoma Type			
POAG	27	21	
PEX	14	17	0.482
Pigmentary	2	0	
LOCS III scale ($NC_1/NC_2/NC_3$)	12/23/6	11/20/7	0.768

LOCS III: lens opacities classification system III; P-ExPress: phaco-ExPress group; P-Trab: phacotrabeculectomy group; * Student's t-test or x^2 test; POAG: primary open-angle glaucoma; PEX: pseudoexfoliation glaucoma.

3.1. Intraocular Pressure

The mean IOP levels before and after surgery are summarized in Table 2.

Table 2. Intraocular pressure (IOP) mean values, median values, standard deviations, and range in the phaco-Ex-Press (P-ExPress) and phaco-trabeculectomy (P-Trab) groups at specific times after surgery.

Time	P-ExPress			P-Trab			P *
	Mean (SD)	Median	Range	Mean (SD)	Median	Range	
Pre-op	25.3 ± 7.1	25.00	12–50	26.8 ± 11.3	25.00	12–62	0.877
1st day	16.7 ± 8.0	16.00	4–29	15.7 ± 7.1	16.00	3–31	0.867
7th day	15.2 ± 6.6	14.00	7–23	16.9 ± 4.8	18.00	3–19	0.236
1st month	17.6 ± 10.2	16.00	8–27	17.3 ± 8.2	16.00	10–26	0.653
3rd month	14.9 ± 3.2	16.00	5–23	14.5 ± 4.1	15.00	7–24	0.645
6th month	15.1 ± 4.3	15.00	7–22	15.9 ± 2.9	16.00	8–23	0.281

P-ExPress: phaco-Ex-Press group; P-Trab: phacotrabeculectomy group; Pre-op: pre-operatively; SD: standard deviation; * Mann-Whitney U test.

3.2. IOP-Lowering Drugs

The average numbers of IOP-lowering medications before and after surgery are summarized in Table 3. In the P-Ex-PRESS and P-Trab groups, two drugs were used before surgery in 20.6% (*n* = 8) and 22.6% (*n* = 8) of patients, respectively. However, during the follow-up, 50% (*n* = 21) and 75% (*n* = 28) of patients were drug-free in the P-Ex-PRESS and P-Trab groups, respectively.

Table 3. Number of hypotensive drugs: mean values, median values, standard deviations, and ranges in the phaco-Ex-Press (P-ExPress) and phaco-trabeculectomy (P-Trab) groups before and 6 months after surgery.

Time	P-ExPress			P-Trab			*p* *
	Mean (SD)	Median	Range	Mean (SD)	Median	Range	
Pre-op	2.91 ± 0.9	3.0	2–4	3.26 ± 0.8	3.0	3–4	0.79
6 mo.	0.46 ± 1	0	-	1.39 ± 1.2	2	0–2	0.3

Pre-op: pre-operatively; mo: months; * Mann–Whitney U test.

3.3. Surgical Success

By the criterion of pressure ≤18 mm Hg, 44% (*n* = 19) and 49% (*n* = 18) of patients achieved complete success in the P-Ex-PRESS and P-Trab groups, respectively (*P* = 0.681). Qualified success was achieved in 63% (*n* = 27) of patients in the P-Ex-PRESS group and 71% (*n* = 27) of patients in the P-Trab group (*P* = 0.561).

3.4. Best-Corrected Visual Acuity

The preoperative and postoperative BCVAs are shown in Table 4.

Table 4. Visual acuity (logMAR) mean values, median values, standard deviations, and ranges in the phaco-ExPress (P-ExPress) and phaco-trabeculectomy (P-Trab) groups before and 6 months after surgery.

Time	P-ExPress			P-Trab			*p* *
	Mean (SD)	Median	Range	Mean (SD)	Median	Range	
Pre-op	0.53 ± 0.55	0.30	0–2.4	0.48 ± 0.5	0.16	0–2	0.68
6 mo.	0.22 ± 0.42	0.1	0–1.7	0.17 ± 0.28	0.05	0–1.4	0.57

mo: months; Pre-op: pre-operatively; SD: standard deviation; * Mann–Whitney U test.

In the P-Ex-PRESS group, BCVA was one line worse in four patients (8.7%). In 12 patients (15.2%), BCVA remained at baseline after surgery and improved from one to nine lines in 61 (76.1%) patients. Vision deterioration due to posterior capsular-bag opacification was noted in one patient. Macular edema caused by chronic hypotension was observed in a single case during the follow-up.

In the P-Trab group, BCVA decreased by one Snellen line in seven patients (8.8%), remained unchanged in six (7.7%), and increased by one to nine lines in 68 (83.5%) patients. The reasons for vision deterioration were posterior capsular-bag opacification, choroidal effusion, and dry age-related macular degeneration.

3.5. Complications and Additional Procedures

Subconjunctival 5-FU injections were administered to nine patients (19.6%) in the P-Ex-PRESS group and nine patients (23.1%) in the P-Trab group (*P* = 0.216). The average dose of 5-FU was 7.0 ± 3.5 mg in the P-Ex-PRESS group (a mean of 1.4 injections per patient) and 8.5 ± 2.3 mg in the P-Trab group (a mean of 1.7 injections) (*P* = 0.105). Needling was used in 11 patients (23.9%) in the P-Ex-PRESS group and in 12 in the P-Trab (30.8%) group (*P* = 0.305). One patient from the P-Ex-PRESS group (2.1%) and two patients from the P-Trab group (5.1%) (*P* = 0.462) underwent laser suturolysis. One patient from the P-Ex-PRESS group (2.3%) was fitted with an additional sealing suture (*P* = 0.354). Two patients from the P-Ex-PRESS group (4.6%) underwent reoperation: one due to extrusion of the mini seton through the scleral flap, and the other due to fibrosis of the filtering bleb. In both cases, classical trabeculectomy was performed. These patients were excluded from the study after the additional surgery, but their previous results were not excluded from the database. One patient from the P-Trab group (2.6%) underwent reoperation due to unsatisfactory IOP regulation. Two patients from the P-ExPress group (4.3%) and one (2.6%) from the P-Trab group had symptoms of malignant glaucoma that occurred at different time-points after surgery and were managed successfully with cycloplegics and compression dressing. The exact rate of complications is shown in Table 5.

Table 5. Complications that were observed in the participants.

	P-ExPress n (%)	P-Trab n (%)	p *
	Intraoperative		
Bleeding	-	1 (2.6)	0.645
	Postoperative		
Hyphema			
blood level in AC	1 (2.1)	1 (2.6)	0.875
erythrocytes in AC	-	-	-
Wound leakage	3 (6.5)	1 (2.6)	0.391
Fibrosis	9 (19.6)	9 (23.1)	0.784
Anterior chamber cells	3 (6.5)	3 (7.7)	0.834
	Hypotony		
until 7 days	-	2 (5.1)	0.115
until 30 days	-	1 (2.6)	0.411
until 180 days	1 (2.1)	1 (2.6)	0.896
Choroid detachment	1 (2.1)	3 (7.7)	0.231
Macular edema	1 (2.1)	-	0.354

AC: anterior chamber; P-ExPress: phaco-Express group; P-Trab: phaco-trabeculectomy, group; * χ^2 test.

3.6. Refractive Analysis of Astigmatism

Arithmetic analysis revealed an astigmatism magnitude of approximately 1 Dcyl in both groups for all analyzed periods. For P-Ex-PRESS, the magnitude was 1.15 ± 0.76 D preoperatively and 0.89 ± 0.52 D postoperatively. For P-Trab, this was 1.13 ± 0.93 D preoperatively and 1.20 ± 0.74 D postoperatively. No differences were found in the magnitude of astigmatism throughout the observation period or between groups (Tables 6 and 7, Figures 1 and 2).

Table 6. Autorefractometry data: mean magnitude of positive cylinder form in the phaco-ExPress (P-ExPress) and phaco-trabeculectomy (P-Trab) groups before and 6 months after surgery.

Time	P-ExPress			P-Trab			p *
	Mean	Median	SD	Mean	Median	SD	
Pre-op	1.15	1.0	0.76	1.13	0.75	0.93	0.175
6 mo.	0.89	0.87	0.52	1.20	1.06	0.75	0.2

mo: months; Pre-op: pre-operatively; * Mann–Whitney U test.

Table 7. Centroids (mean astigmatism with its axis) and direction of astigmatism in the phaco-ExPress (P-ExPress) and phaco-trabeculectomy (P-Trab) groups before and 6 months after surgery.

Time	P-ExPress			P-Trab			p *
	Centroid	Axis	Trend	Centroid	Axis	Trend	
Pre-op	0.44	177.42	ATR	0.16	140.61	OBLIQUE	0.5
6 mo.	0.35	7.71	ATR	0.39	29.47	OBLIQUE	0.38

ATR: Against-the-rule; * Mann–Whitney U test.

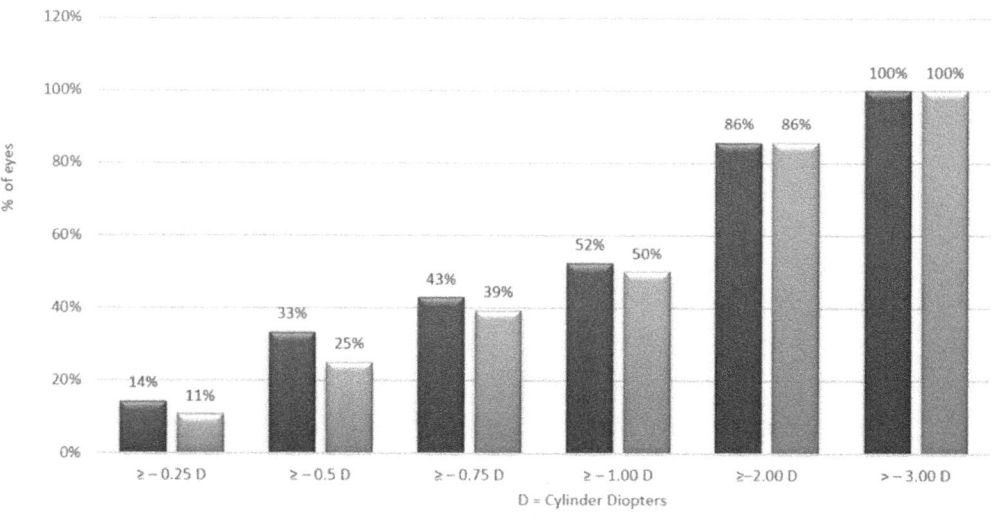

Figure 1. Cumulative values of astigmatism in the P-Trab group.

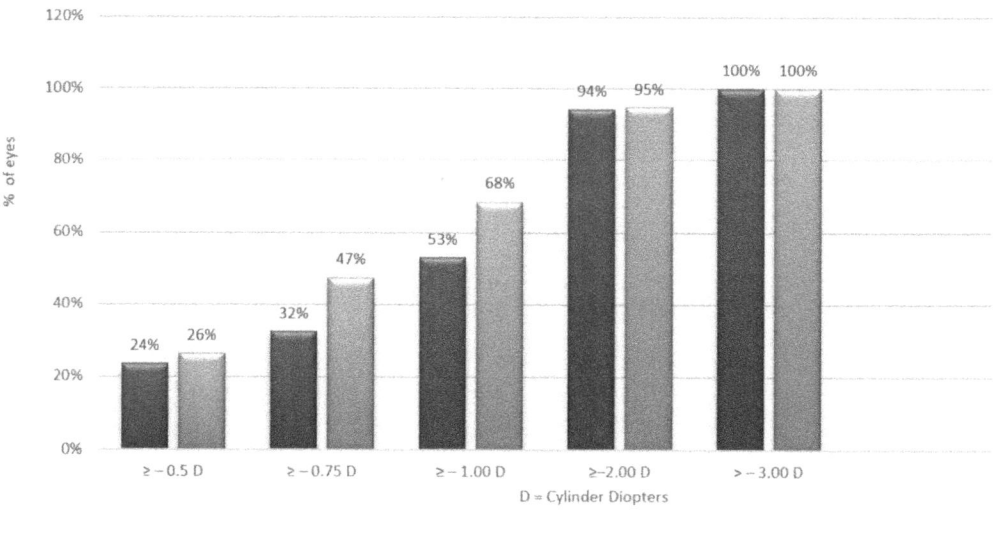

Figure 2. Cumulative values of astigmatism in the P-Ex-PRESS group.

3.7. Vector Analysis of Astigmatism

The mean values of astigmatism and the corresponding axes are presented numerically in Table 7 and graphically in centroid form on double-angle plots in Figures 3 and 4.

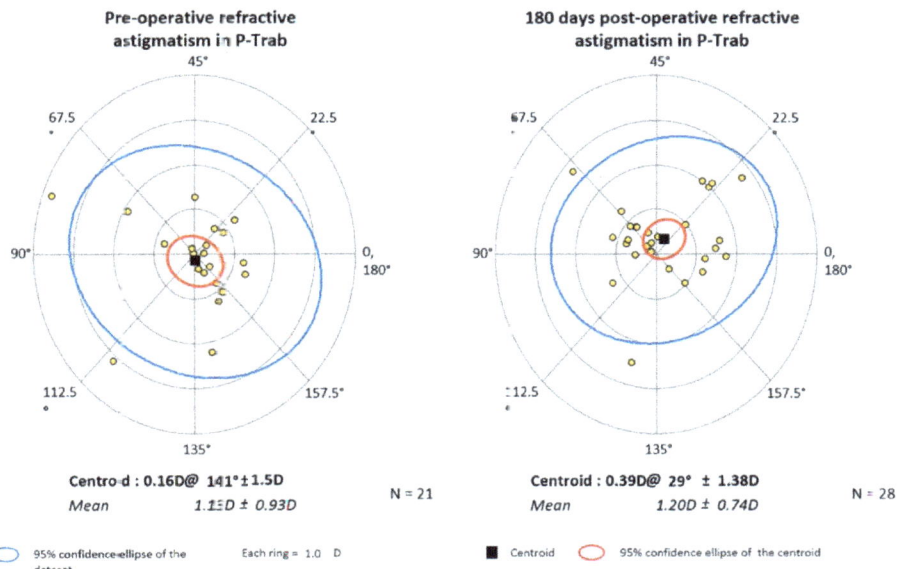

Figure 3. The mean values of astigmatism, with the axes, presented in centroid form on double angle plots for the P-Trab group (The black square indicates the centroid. The red circle indicates the 95% confidence ellipse of the centroid. The blue circle indicates the 95% confidence ellipse of the dataset. Yellow dots indicate individual values of astigmatism. Each ring indicates 1.0 D. Astigmatism trend in P-trab is oblique before and after the surgery).

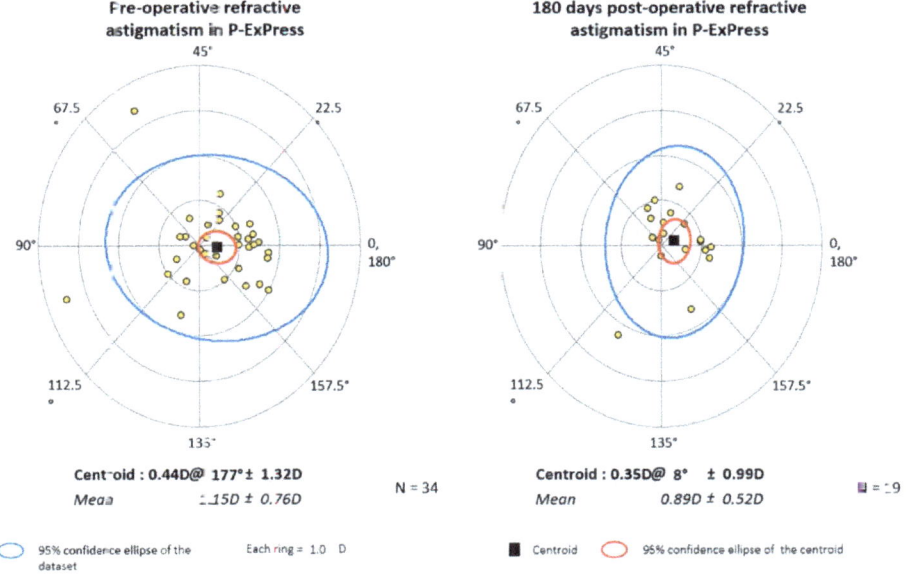

Figure 4. The mean values of astigmatism, with the axes, presented in centroid form on double angle plots for the P-Ex-PRESS group (The black square indicates the centroid. The red circle indicates the 95% confidence ellipse of the centroid. The blue circle indicates the 95% confidence ellipse of the dataset. Yellow dots indicate individual values of astigmatism. Each ring indicates 1.0 D. In P-Ex-PRESS astigmatism trend it is against the rule before and after surgery.

4. Discussion

To the best of our knowledge, this is the first prospective study to compare P-Trab and combined phaco-Ex-PRESS device implantation based on SIA in glaucoma patients. Surprisingly, despite the use of different surgical techniques, the procedures did not differ when determining SIA. We also evaluated the postoperative complications of surgery and analyzed the IOP-lowering effect of combined surgeries.

In this study, astigmatism was of the ATR type in the P-Ex-PRESS group, and the direction had not changed by the 6-month follow-up. Astigmatism values changed slightly during the follow-up period, dropping from an average of 1.15 D to 0.89 D ($P > 0.05$). In the analyzed P-Trab group, mean astigmatism was 0.86 D before surgery and increased to 1.26 D after surgery ($P > 0.05$). Both before and after surgery, the direction of astigmatism was oblique.

Our study showed that despite the use of different surgical instruments and the discrepancy in the extend of tissue excision, astigmatism does not differ between the groups. These findings may confirm the assertion of Hugkulstone [6] that the astigmatism shift originates from a surgically induced gape around the scleral flap or the number of flap sutures (which were the same in both groups) and not from the removal of tissue under the scleral flap that leaves the corneal edge unsupported (which differed our groups); however, owing to the elasticity of the human sclera, this might be irrelevant for postoperative BCVA.

Our results contradict the findings of Tanito et al., who found in a retrospective study significant differences in SIA occur due to trabeculectomy and those due to ExPress implant trabeculotomy ab externo and microhook ab interno trabeculotomy. As expected, they found the least SIA after the minimally invasive procedures [14].

To date, the results of previous studies on the magnitude and direction of SIA are inconsistent. Hammel et al. [15] analyzed changes in corneal curvature with a Pentacam after implanting an Ex-PRESS [14]. On the first postoperative day, the anterior corneal astigmatism increased from 2.6 ± 3.3 to 4.7 ± 3.1 D ($P = 0.19$), but the curvature of the posterior cornea also changed (0.4 to 0.9). However, the changes were not statistically significant after 3 months. They observed a non-significant correlation between the increase in astigmatism and the presence of a low IOP due to anti-glaucoma surgery, which was also previously reported by Razeghinejad [16]. Hornová reported that ATR astigmatism was 0.8 D at 6 months after trabeculectomy [17]. Claridge et al. found statistically insignificant ATR astigmatism in some patients and statistically significant WTR in others [9]. They showed that the major change in the astigmatism vector was 1.25 ± 1.08 after 6 months in the vertical meridian. The authors assumed that vertical steepening was due to significant tissue contraction caused by excessive cauterization of the sclera. They also suspected that a large filtration cushion and postoperative ptosis could provoke vertical corneal steepening.

Law et al. compared the refractive results after P-Trab and phaco alone [18]. No differences between the expected and achieved refraction after surgery were observed, despite changes in corneal curvature and eyeball length. In their study, the average size of the cylinder after anti-glaucoma surgery was 1.31 ± 0.86 D, which was slightly larger than that in the control group, where the induced astigmatism was 0.44. There was a tendency towards short-sightedness, caused by shortening the eyeball length after trabeculectomy, as well as after implantation of drainage valves [19].

Cunliffe et al. performed tests on 19 eyes after trabeculectomy and evaluated the refraction and keratometry data [20]. Their findings included a reduction in the vertical corneal radius, and therefore a trend of astigmatism towards WTR in the early postoperative period. They proposed that the change in astigmatism was due to sclerostomy healing, causing the corneal edge to contract during trabeculectomy, resulting in a reduction of the horizontal corneal radius. After 2 months, the corneal radius returned to its preoperative value, probably due to a decrease in suture tension on the scleral flap. In addition, they noticed changes in anterior segment parameters, with the refraction shift toward myopia reaching 2 D. The hypothesis of a decrease in suture tone on the scleral flap does not coincide with the observations reported by Lima et al. [21], who did not observe an effect of laser suturolysis on the corneal curvature; however, they observed a shift in astigmatism in the direction of WTR of between 1.5 and 2.5 D, which persisted up to 3 months after surgery. They reported that changes in keratometry were underestimated compared to topography findings.

Our study has a few limitations. First, the data used for calculations were from autorefractometry and represented whole astigmatism, including lenticular astigmatism preoperatively and IOL postoperatively. In contrast, clinicians are concerned about overall astigmatism because it affects postoperative visual acuity. Second, a comparative study with keratometry could not be conducted, because the keratometry data were incomplete. Third, staff that performed the follow-up visits was not blinded; BCVA and IOP were measured with knowledge of the surgery that had been performed. Another limitation is the 6-month follow-up time. Existing data on astigmatism after anti-glaucoma surgery is inconsistent. According to one study, changes in corneal curvature after surgery can last up to 12 months [6]. Other studies have reported that such changes disappear after 6 months [7], and others found that refraction was constant after 2 to 3 months [22].

In future studies, blinding of all investigators could improve the reliability of the outcome data. Also, cornea mapping should be obtained before and after surgery to permit an exact assessment of the astigmatism. Another issue for future investigations is assessment of the possible impact of the Ex-PRESS device (among the other implants) on endothelial cell loss.

5. Conclusions

In conclusion, the P-Ex-PRESS and P-Trab procedures did not differ in inducing postoperative astigmatism or refractive errors; the astigmatism trend noted during observation remained the same in both groups (ATR in P-Ex-PRESS and oblique in P-Trab). Comparable results were found in the groups for final visual acuity. The two procedures showed similar antihypertensive efficacy in treating open-angle glaucoma. This study confirms the noninferiority of the Ex-PRESS device, which is relevant when making optimal clinical decisions with patients, as Ex-PRESS is comparatively less invasive than trabeculectomy.

Author Contributions: J.K. worked on the main text. A.B. worked on figures, and methodology, E.S. collected data from patients and worked on the main text, Z.M. reviewed whole article, M.R. worked on the main text, and also analyzed and interpreted the data. All authors have read and agreed to the published version of the manuscript.

Funding: This research received no external funding.

Institutional Review Board Statement: The study was conducted according to the guidelines of the Declaration of Helsinki, and approved by the Ethics Committee of Medical University of Bialystok, Poland (16/UMB/2014).

Informed Consent Statement: Informed consent was obtained from all subjects involved in the study.

Data Availability Statement: All materials and information are available upon e-mail request to the corresponding author. The names and exact data of the study participants may not be available because of privacy policies.

Conflicts of Interest: The authors declare no conflict of interest.

References

1. Traverso, C.E.; De Feo, F.; Messas-Kaplan, A.; Denis, P.; Levartovsky, S.; Sellem, E.; Badalà, F.; Zagorski, Z.; Bron, A.; Gandolfi, S.; et al. Long term effect on IOP of a stainless steel glaucoma drainage implant (Ex-PRESS) in combined surgery with phacoemulsification. *Br. J. Ophthalmol.* **2005**, *89*, 425–429. [CrossRef] [PubMed]
2. Netland, P.A.; Sarkisian, S.R.; Moster, M.R.; Ahmed, I.I.; Condor, G.; Salim, S.; Sherwood, M.B.; Siegfried, C.J. Randomized, prospective, comparative trial of EX-PRESS glaucoma filtration device versus trabeculectomy (XVT study). *Am. J. Ophthalmol.* **2014**, *157*, 433–440.e5. [CrossRef] [PubMed]
3. Tzu, J.H.; Shah, C.T.; Galor, A.; Junk, A.K.; Sastry, A.; Wellik, S.R. Refractive outcomes of combined cataract and glaucoma surgery. *J. Glaucoma* **2015**, *24*, 161–164. [CrossRef]

4. Chan, H.H.L.; Kong, Y.X.G. Glaucoma surgery and induced astigmatism: A systematic review. *Eye Vis. (Lond.)* **2017**, *4*, 27. [CrossRef] [PubMed]
5. Moschos, M.M.; Chatziralli, I.P.; Tsatsos, M. One-site versus two-site phacotrabeculectomy: A prospective randomized study. *Clin. Interv. Aging* **2015**, *10*, 1393–1399. [CrossRef] [PubMed]
6. Hugkulstone, C.E. Changes in keratometry following trabeculectomy. *Br. J. Ophthalmol.* **1991**, *75*, 217–218. [CrossRef]
7. Cravy, T.V. Calculation of the change in corneal astigmatism following cataract extraction. *Ophthalmic Surg.* **1979**, *10*, 38–49.
8. Cashwell, L.F.; Martin, C.A. Axial length decrease accompanying successful glaucoma filtration surgery. *Ophthalmology* **1999**, *106*, 2307–2311. [CrossRef]
9. Claridge, K.G.; Galbraith, J.K.; Karmel, V.; Bates, A.K. The effect of trabeculectomy on refraction, keratometry and corneal topography. *Eye (Lond.)* **1995**, *9*, 292–298. [CrossRef]
10. Park, S.H.; Park, K.H.; Kim, J.M.; Choi, C.Y. Relation between axial length and ocular parameters. *Ophthalmologica* **2010**, *224*, 188–193. [CrossRef]
11. Stawowski, Ł.; Konopińska, J.; Deniziak, M.; Saeed, E.; Zalewska, R.; Mariak, Z. Comparison of ExPress mini-device implantation alone or combined with phacoemulsification for the treatment of open-angle glaucoma. *J. Ophthalmol.* **2015**, *2015*, 613280. [CrossRef] [PubMed]
12. Byszewska, A.; Konopińska, J.; Kicińska, A.K.; Mariak, Z.; Rękas, M. Canaloplasty in the treatment of primary open-angle glaucoma: Patient selection and perspectives. *Clin. Ophthalmol.* **2019**, *13*, 2617–2629. [CrossRef] [PubMed]
13. Holladay, J.T.; Maverick, K.J. Relationship of the actual thick intraocular lens optic to the thin lens equivalent. *Am. J. Ophthalmol.* **1998**, *126*, 339–347. [CrossRef]
14. Tanito, M.; Matsuzaki, Y.; Ikeda, Y.; Fujihara, E. Comparison of surgically induced astigmatism following different glaucoma operations. *Clin. Ophthalmol.* **2017**, *11*, 2113–2120. [CrossRef]
15. Hammel, N.; Lusky, M.; Kaiserman, I.; Robinson, A.; Bahar, I. Changes in anterior segment parameters after insertion of Ex-PRESS miniature glaucoma implant. *J. Glaucoma* **2013**, *22*, 565–568. [CrossRef]
16. Razeghinejad, M.R.; Dehghani, C. Effect of ocular hypotony secondary to cyclodialysis cleft on corneal topography. *Cornea* **2008**, *27*, 609–611. [CrossRef]
17. Hornová, J. Trabeculectomy with releasable sutures and corneal topography. *Ceske Slov. Oftalmol.* **1998**, *54*, 368–372.
18. Law, S.K.; Mansury, A.M.; Vasudev, D.; Caprioli, J. Effects of combined cataract surgery and trabeculectomy with mitomycin C on ocular dimensions. *Br. J. Ophthalmol.* **2005**, *89*, 1021–1025. [CrossRef]
19. Francis, B.A.; Wang, M.; Lei, H.; Du, L.T.; Minckler, D.S.; Green, R.L.; Roland, C. Changes in axial length following trabeculectomy and glaucoma drainage device surgery. *Br. J. Ophthalmol.* **2005**, *89*, 17–20. [CrossRef]
20. Cunliffe, I.A.; Dapling, R.B.; West, J.; Longstaff, S. A prospective study examining the changes in factors that affect visual acuity following trabeculectomy. *Eye (Lond.)* **1992**, *6*, 618–622. [CrossRef]
21. Lima, V.C.; Prata, T.S.; Castro, D.P.; Castro, L.C.; De Moraes, C.G.; Mattox, C.; Rosen, R.B.; Liebmann, J.M.; Ritch, R. Macular changes detected by Fourier-domain optical coherence tomography in patients with hypotony without clinical maculopathy. *Acta Ophthalmol.* **2011**, *89*, e274–e277. [CrossRef] [PubMed]
22. Delbeke, H.; Stalmans, I.; Vandewalle, E.; Zeyen, T. The effect of trabeculectomy on astigmatism. *J. Glaucoma* **2016**, *25*, e308–e312. [CrossRef] [PubMed]

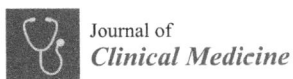

Review
Treatment of Glaucoma Patients with Flammer Syndrome

Katarzyna Konieczka * and Josef Flammer

Department of Ophthalmology, University of Basel, 4056 Basel, Switzerland; josef.flammer@unibas.ch
* Correspondence: katarzyna.konieczka@usb.ch; Tel.: +41-612-658-803

Abstract: Flammer syndrome (FS) describes a phenotype characterized by the presence of primary vascular dysregulation along with a number of symptoms and signs. Although most people with FS are healthy, FS favors the occurrence of certain diseases, such as normal tension glaucoma. This is because disturbed autoregulation makes the eye more sensitive to intraocular pressure (IOP) spikes or blood pressure drops. Treatment of FS is generally appropriate when patients either suffer greatly from their symptoms or if we can assume that it has contributed to a disease. In glaucoma, this may be the case if the glaucoma damage progresses despite well-controlled IOP. Both the still sparse scientific studies and our long clinical experience suggest that FS-targeted therapy not only relieves the symptoms of FS but also slows the progression of glaucoma damage in selected cases. This description is intended not only to help affected patients but to also motivate clinicians and researchers to conduct therapy studies to confirm or refute our observations.

Keywords: glaucoma; normal tension glaucoma; Flammer syndrome; calcium channel blockers; magnesium; nutrition; antioxidants

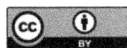

Citation: Konieczka, K.; Flammer, J. Treatment of Glaucoma Patients with Flammer Syndrome. *J. Clin. Med* **2021**, *10*, 4227. https://doi.org/10.3390/jcm10184227

Academic Editor: Georgios Labiris

Received: 16 August 2021
Accepted: 13 September 2021
Published: 17 September 2021

Publisher's Note: MDPI stays neutral with regard to jurisdictional claims in published maps and institutional affiliations.

Copyright: © 2021 by the authors. Licensee MDPI, Basel, Switzerland. This article is an open access article distributed under the terms and conditions of the Creative Commons Attribution (CC BY) license (https://creativecommons.org/licenses/by/4.0/).

1. Introduction

Flammer syndrome (FS) [1–5] describes a phenotype characterized by the presence of primary vascular dysregulation [3,6] together with a combination of symptoms and signs that result from predisposition to generally increased sensitivity. The main focus is a modified, mostly increased response of the blood vessels to certain stimuli, such as cold or emotional stress, and the resulting phenomenon, such as cold hands. This combination of symptoms was first primarily observed in patients, especially those with normal tension glaucoma (NTG). Later, we noticed that the same combination of symptoms can also occur in healthy people but less frequently and usually less pronounced [1,3]. Therefore, we created a multiple-choice questionnaire that patients can fill out prior to consultation [5,7].

FS is not a disease but rather a predisposition that usually does not require treatment. However, treatment is recommended if diseases fostered by FS arise [7,8] or if people subjectively suffer from their symptoms. Although the syndrome is quite prevalent, there have only been a few studies dealing with the therapy. In contrast, there are many years of clinical experience. Therefore, the following recommendations are based on both studies and clinical experience. Although most people with FS are healthy and FS even seems to protect against atherosclerosis, it is a risk factor for some other diseases [8]. Here, we focus on glaucoma [3,6,7,9], specifically NTG [7].

Some recommendations concerning lifestyle management, nutrition, and drug therapy that have proven helpful in our clinical glaucoma practice are discussed here.

2. What Should Patients with FS Avoid?

Patients with FS generally observe themselves well, and they know what is good and what is not good for them. Nevertheless, they are usually grateful and relieved when their doctor discusses the following aspects.

2.1. Cold Exposure

Cold hands and/or feet are a leading symptom of FS [10]. That is why people with FS generally prefer to avoid the cold, and they often notice that they can fall asleep sooner if they warm up their feet or wear socks to bed. Others report symptoms such as chest pain when they drink cold liquids. While this is usually harmless, cold can also be dangerous in rare cases.

We were treating a FS patient with NTG who noticed a sudden increase in her visual field defect while skiing in very cold weather. The perimetry on the very next day revealed a new, large absolute scotoma.

Two female NTG patients independent of each other fell unconscious after jumping into the cold waters of the North Sea. Both ladies had to be rescued by their partners, and this happened twice to one of them. A young doctor with pronounced FS suffered a heart attack when he jumped into a cold swimming pool.

These clinical observations have also been confirmed by experimental studies [11,12]. The visual fields of glaucoma patients with FS temporarily worsened when they put one hand in cold water, while the visual fields of patients without FS remained stable [12].

2.2. Psychological Stress

Everybody experiences emotional stress from time to time, which can trigger a variety of different physical symptoms. In people with FS, these symptoms are mostly vascular. For instance, they notice cold hands or white and red spots on their face or neck [1,13].

Using thermographic images, we have observed that, in people with FS, some areas of the face cool down while other areas warm up at the same time during emotional stress.

A very successful young musician suffered from an NTG. During capillary microscopy of the nailfold, the cold provocation caused a blood flow standstill of 60 s. Later, when she told about her problems with her husband, the blood flow stopped for 130 s.

These symptoms and signs in the fingers are harmless. If, however, these phenomena occur in other organs, such as the eye, it can potentially cause damage.

One of our NTG patients with FS was stable for years, but within a three-month period, her visual field deteriorated very much. Only when we asked her specifically about stress did she describe heavy burden because of her daughter's divorce.

Three independent bankers with FS had developed an anterior ischemic optic neuropathy (AION). Two of them became sick during the great financial crisis of 2008 and the third individual became so later but also after he lost money in the stock market.

Another young patient with FS had an argument with her superior. She developed an AION in her left eye on the same day and was treated in an emergency center with corticosteroids. They were ineffective, and she became blind in her affected left eye. Three months later, under similar conditions, she noticed visual disturbances in her right eye and visited our clinic. We diagnosed a fresh AION in her right eye and immediately initiated a full FS therapy (see below). Her visual field, visual acuity, and optic nerve head recovered. Today, many years later, this right eye is still healthy.

A man with FS in his mid-50s lost his job. On the same day on his way home, he caused a car accident. He was sent to a hospital with minor injuries. However, when he arrived at the hospital, he noticed that he could not see anything in one eye. An AION was diagnosed, but unfortunately, he was not transferred to us until a few days later. He remained blind in this eye.

An older teacher at a high school who had already lost one eye to an AION some years earlier had an argument with the parents of one of his pupils. That same evening, he developed an AION in his remaining good eye. Fortunately, we had the opportunity to start treatment the same evening, and his eye largely recovered. Today, many years later, the man is retired and is subjectively not disturbed by his visual field deficits and can read well with this eye. His FS symptoms have decreased.

A monk with FS was treated for an AION. A few weeks later, similar symptoms appeared in his other eye, and he finally came to us. We found a massive increase in retinal venous pressure (RVP), a phenomenon we often observe in FS patients [14,15]. After we decreased the RVP (see below), the first eye improved slightly and the second eye improved significantly.

Another man with FS and an advanced NTG felt significant pressure to perform in his job as a goldsmith. He took early retirement, and his FS symptoms subsided for the most part and the glaucoma stabilized.

A 14-year-old FS girl was under tremendous stress because she could not meet her school's expectations. She developed an AION, and unfortunately, we did not see her until two weeks after the event. She remained blind in one eye, but her other eye has remained healthy for many years now with mild prophylactic therapy.

A young man with FS was responsible for the maintenance and repair of postbuses. One day, chips were introduced to acknowledge workers' individual achievements. This put him under massive psychological and emotional pressure, and he developed a central serous chorioretinopathy [16,17]. An indocyanine green angiography revealed a distinct venous dysregulation in the choroid of the affected eye and, to a lesser extent, also in the unaffected eye. The patient completely recovered after he changed his job.

Even more frequently than AION, we have seen retinal vein occlusions after stress in otherwise completely healthy people with FS, including doctors in our hospital and professors from our university. A young sportswoman developed very high RVP up to a venous stasis retinopathy after breaking up with her boyfriend, but she recovered slowly once treatment was administered (see below). In another researcher, otherwise healthy, we also observed increased RVP when she realized she was going to lose her job at the university.

A student from a developing country was studying in Switzerland. He came under enormous stress because he was afraid that he would have to leave Switzerland before he could finish his studies. Three months after subjective visual disturbances, he was diagnosed with NTG with a new onset scotoma in the visual field.

Of course, stress simply cannot be avoided. However, it is possible to manage private and professional life in such a way that stress becomes less pronounced. There are also strategies, such as autogenic training and yoga, that can help a person deal with unavoidable stress. Sometimes professional support is needed, and if potentially dangerous vascular reactions persist, prophylactic drug therapy may make sense (see below).

2.3. Extreme Physical Activity

Exercise is healthy for everybody, including people with FS, as long as it is not too extreme. As we have observed that people with outdoor job suffer much less frequently from both FS symptoms and FS-associated diseases than people with indoor jobs [3,18], we recommend exercising and/or playing sports outdoors as often as possible. We have also observed that exposure to daylight reduces FS symptoms. With this in mind, we recommend exercising or playing sports outside during the day instead of inside or at night.

Occasionally, we have observed patients who exercise intensively for long periods without interruption, and some almost become addicted to it. Many FS patients jog or cycle very intensively. Reducing these extreme activities usually improves vascular regulation.

A young man with FS and advanced NTG rode his bike for several hours every day in a mountain area because he felt he needed it. While monitoring his blood pressure (BP) over a 24 h period, his systolic BP dropped to 65 mm Hg at night and sometimes dropped even lower. We recommended that he shorten his trips to about one hour a day. Fortunately, his nighttime BP dropped less and his glaucoma stabilized.

Patients with FS are also more sensitive to vibrations [3,4,18].

A young woman with FS noticed a slight earthquake, while other people in her environment did not notice it. Vibrations of the hands can lead to vasoconstrictions, and such individuals should not work with compressors. They are also more sensitive to mechanical traction. It is very common for FS patients to require more treatment and recovery time after whiplash injury.

2.4. Rapid Increase in Altitude

The response to lower oxygen concentrations at higher elevations is stronger in FS subjects than in individuals without FS, and they take longer to adapt to the condition.

A young lady with FS treated for a venous stasis retinopathy fell unconscious on a hot air balloon ride over the Alps. She regained consciousness immediately after the balloon dropped to a lower elevation.

A young FS man took a cable car from 1500 to 3200 m above sea level. He was unconscious when he arrived, so he was immediately taken back to the valley by gondola where he quickly recovered.

In a flight simulator study, we found that young healthy FS subjects were less able to tolerate reduced atmospheric pressure. For some of them, it was so bad that they had to abort the study, while subjects without FS tolerated it very well.

3. Nutritional Recommendations for Patients with FS

While most dietary advice is rightly aimed at reducing body weight, people with FS should make sure that their body mass index (BMI) does not fall too low. The lower a person's BMI, the more intense the FS symptoms. A normal body weight should be aimed. Because fasting can exacerbate the symptoms of FS, we advise patients with FS against prolonged or intensive fasting [19].

Glaucoma patients with FS have increased oxidative stress [20,21], particularly in the mitochondria of neural axons. Food should therefore contain as many natural antioxidants, for example polyphenols, as possible. [22,23]. Please also refer to Section 4.2.9.

An increase in omega-3 fatty acids, especially in the form of seafood, can be helpful. It reduces FS symptoms by upregulating the uncoupling proteins, thereby increasing ATP-independent heat production.

Although the magnesium (Mg) plasma concentration in FS patients is usually normal, the diet should contain sufficient Mg. An Mg supplement is discussed below.

FS patients often have very low BP. While reduction of salt intake is generally rightly recommended, particularly for patients with arterial hypertension, FS patients with severe arterial hypotension should consume enough salt, especially in the evening, to avoid major drops in BP during sleep.

People with FS also have reduced feeling of thirst, which often leaves them dehydrated. Therefore, it is important that they make sure that they drink enough fluids, also in the evening before going to sleep.

4. Drug Treatment of Patients with FS

Of course, we only treat FS if necessary, and this is especially true for drug therapy. As ophthalmologists, we treat FS patients with eye diseases such as glaucoma (particularly NTG), retinal vein occlusions despite the lack of classical risk factors, and central serous chorioretinopathy. However, it is important to emphasize that FS does not only affect the eye [3,8,24]. Many of our patients or their relatives have also experienced nonocular diseases associated with FS, such as acute hearing loss, heart attacks despite lacking classical risk factors, certain autoimmune diseases, etc. [3,8]. The therapy that we employ is administered in a holistic manner, and we do not treat just one organ such as the eye.

In glaucoma, we primarily lower the intraocular pressure (IOP). This also makes sense for glaucoma patients with FS. FS patients usually have disturbed autoregulation and are therefore more sensitive to IOP peaks and BP dips. Often, however, IOP reduction and IOP stabilization alone are not sufficient. These are especially the cases in which we recommend treatment of FS.

4.1. Drug Sensitivity

Patients with FS often tell us that they cannot tolerate certain medications very well or apparently not at all in some cases and therefore prefer herbal remedies or homeopathic therapy. Based on our experience, however, these patients can actually tolerate these drugs if we prescribe much smaller doses than normal, which can be up to 10 times lower. Interestingly, the main effect usually remains, but the side effects disappear.

We draw the attention of patients with FS to the fact that their children are also more likely to have FS. The 18-year-old son of one of our NTG patients with FS was hospitalized at an internal medicine clinic due to general infection. During the stay, his BP dropped so low that he had to be given adrenaline intravenously. The resulting vasoconstrictive reaction was so violent that he lost fingers, toes, and the tip of his nose.

We recommend that FS patients start drug treatment at a very low dose whenever possible and then increase it slowly until they see the desired effect or until side effects occur. We recommend that a person with FS should be particularly cautious with all vasoconstrictive medications. Often, neither the doctors nor the patients notice that many different medications (e.g., some psychotropic drugs) have a vasoconstrictive side effect.

Based on our experience and also published information, surgery and especially anesthesia should be carefully planned for FS patients [25,26].

We investigated the effect of glaucoma drugs on corneal temperature. After one drop of brimonidine, the temperature of the cornea dropped for approximately 90 min due to the vasoconstrictive effect of brimonidine [27], whereas we observed no cooling under placebo. Interestingly, this effect was significantly stronger in patients with FS than in patients without FS (CTR NCT01201551, publication in preparation). Our glaucoma patients with FS generally did not tolerate brimonidine very well compared to patients without FS.

The symptoms of FS decrease significantly within a few years after menopause, and NTG thus usually (but not always) stabilizes. If women take postmenopausal hormone therapy that contains estrogen, both the FS symptoms and the glaucoma can worsen again. In case of doubt, the regulation of the eye blood circulation can be measured before and after the beginning of therapy.

4.2. Pharmaceutical Improvement of Regulation of the Microcirculation

Primary vascular dysregulation [3,6], the core component of FS, has not been known for very long. It is therefore not surprising that there are only a few types of drugs available, and the number of clinical studies is limited. Unfortunately, the pharmaceutical industry has hardly addressed this issue until now. Nevertheless, we are already able to effectively help these patients. We have had good experience with calcium channel blockers and magnesium.

4.2.1. Calcium Channel Blockers (CCBs)

In ex vivo studies, we have demonstrated that CCBs significantly reduce the effect of endothelin-1 (ET) in ocular circulation [28,29]. In FS patients, we found a slight increase in plasma levels of ET [30]. However, even more important was our observation that the lower the BP, the greater the ET sensitivity in these patients [31].

Even before we knew this rational justification for CCB treatment, we already had clinical experience with it [5]. The positive visual field response to CCBs in certain patients was one of the cornerstones of discovering primary vascular dysregulation and FS. We have conducted various visual field studies. Over time, we noticed that it was always the same patients who showed a visual field response, whether it was an improvement under caroboanhydrase inhibitors [32], CCBs [33], and CO_2 respiration [34] or a worsening caused by cold provocation [12]. Moreover, the visual field response occurred in the same patients who also showed prolonged arrest in blood circulation of the nailfold after cold provocation and shortening of this arrest after CCBs. Controversial discussions regarding the benefits associated with CCBs began to surface, particularly for glaucoma patients [35]. We had to clear up a lot of misunderstandings. First of all, we cannot simply expect a positive outcome in all patients, treatment only works if primary vascular dysregulation or FS is actually present. There were also fears of a "steal effect", which means that the vessels in healthy areas would be dilated, so even less blood would flow in the diseased areas. However, this is unlikely as such a steal effect would hardly explain visual field improvements, and it became evident that CCBs dilate pathologically contracted blood vessels more than healthy ones.

Others feared that CCBs would lower the BP of such patients even further and that this would be dangerous, particularly for glaucoma patients. We address this risk based on the following considerations: (a) we use very low doses that hardly ever lower BP; (b) the BP lowering effect of CCB is either small or nonexistent in patients who already have low BP; (c) animal experiments have shown that nifedipine increases ocular blood flow, even when it reduces BP [36]; and (d) if the ocular perfusion would decrease, we would not observe stabilization or even improvement but rather a deterioration of the visual field.

Others have assumed that fat-soluble (centrally acting) CCBs (e.g., nimodipine) would be better than water-soluble (peripherally acting) CCBs, such as nifedipine. This applies to diseases of the brain and retina as long as the blood-brain or blood-retina barrier is intact. For glaucoma, however, we have had the opposite experience, which may be explained by the fact that there is actually no blood-brain barrier in the optic nerve head [23]. It is important to note that studies comparing different CCBs in glaucoma patients are yet to be undertaken. In very severe cases, such as acute AION in FS patients, we start with a combination of nifedipine with nimodipine and then stop the nifedipine after a few days.

Under normal condition, we start with 1 mg nifedipine (i.e., 1 drop of a nifedipine solution) orally per day and then slowly increase the dose to 2, 3, or more mg depending on the patient, the BP, and the disease we are targeting. As nifedipine has a short half-life, patients dilute it in a liquid of their choice and drink it throughout the day. Because nifedipine is sensitive to light, we recommend using a light-protected bottle or keeping it in the dark (e.g., in the refrigerator or cabinet).

Fortunately, the half-life of the effect is significantly longer than the half-life of the blood level. Intake during the day instead of at night is desirable as thermographic studies have revealed that FS patients have vascular dysregulation during the day but not when they are asleep.

Many doctors hardly believe that such low doses could have an effect. Let us illustrate this by example. A researcher working for a pharmaceutical company in Basel told us about the fate of her father who lived in a developing country. He was diagnosed with NTG, and his ophthalmologist noticed a fast progression since he was on dialysis. In addition, the patient noticed a temporary deterioration in his vision after dialysis. Unfortunately, it was not possible for him to travel to us for an examination. We have observed similar events in patients on dialysis. They all had increased ET levels in the blood, which resulted in increased RVP, which contributed to progression of glaucoma damage. Assuming a similar situation, we recommended a therapy with a relatively low dose of nifedipine. A few weeks later, we received a letter from the patient informing us that his vision had improved and that his visual field deficits had decreased after the initiation of 1 and then 2 mg of nifedipine per day.

If a higher dose is necessary or desired, we replace nifedipine with amlodipine (5 mg once a day). Amlodipine has effects that are similar to nifedipine, but it has a longer half-life. However, unfortunately, it is only available in doses of 5 mg or higher.

Although FS patients usually have rather low BP, some of them develop high BP in old age. In such cases, we recommend an antihypertensive treatment containing a low dose of a CCB (e.g., a combination of an ACE inhibitor with 5 mg amlodipine).

We know that ET increases RVP [37], but not every high RVP is ET induced. Accordingly, one cannot lower every RVP with nifedipine. In addition, CCBs, and thus nifedipine, only inhibit ET-induced influx of calcium from the outside into the cell but not ET-induced release of calcium from the cell's internal storage. This means that we can reduce but not completely eliminate the effect of ET. In addition, the venous resistance that leads to the increase in RVP does not always occur at the level of the optic disc. This can also be further in the retina or deeper in the optic nerve. In such cases, CCBs that are less water soluble, such as nimodipine, help better.

CCBs have the well-known effect of lowering blood pressure and side effects such as flush or ankle edema. However, as we prescribe extremely low doses (much lower than usually prescribed by internists), we see such side effects extremely rarely. Nevertheless, to be on the safe side, we recommend 24 h blood measurement before and after starting therapy with low-dose CCB.

4.2.2. Endothelin Blockers

Endothelin blockers are particularly interesting [38]. Unfortunately, the benefit for FS subjects has not yet been investigated in detail, and they are not yet approved for this application. However, we know that RVP is mainly regulated by ET and that ET blockers reduce increased RVP [39]. Endothelin traps and the delivery of artificial transcription factors are also under investigation [40].

4.2.3. Magnesium

Magnesium (Mg) is a physiological CCB. We have shown that Mg reduces the effect of ET both in vitro and in ex vivo [41]. We have further observed a slight improvement in the visual field of glaucoma patients with FS [42]. Mg has only mild side effects, such as diarrhea, which disappears after reducing the dose. Often, it is better tolerated by taking it together with yoghurt. We normally use 10–20 mmol of Mg per day, but there are only a few studies in the available literature and the effect is relatively small. We normally start treatment with Mg, and if the effect is insufficient, we combine it with a low dose of CCB.

4.2.4. Betaxolol

Studies have demonstrated that glaucoma patients treated with betaxolol have a smaller rate of visual field deterioration than patients treated with timolol despite the fact that betaxolol reduces IOP less than timolol [43]. This can be explained by a slight calcium channel blocking effect of betaxolol. As betaxolol is beta-1 specific, it is generally tolerated by most (but not all) FS patients.

4.2.5 Triflusal

Triflusal is a compound related to aspirin. However, in contrast to aspirin, it leaves the arachidonic acid pathway intact, favors the production of nitric oxide (NO), and increases the concentration of cyclic nucleotide in endothelial cells, which results in peripheral vasodilatation [44]. We do not have much experience with it because it is not yet on the market in Switzerland.

4.2.6. Propranolol

Propranolol is a beta-blocker as well as a weak CCB. Taking very low doses (5–10 mg per day) for days or weeks help some FS patients when emotional stress is unavoidable and causes symptoms.

4.2.7. Carbonic Anhydrase Inhibitors (CAI)

Acetazolamide is used to reduce both IOP and intracranial pressure. It also dilatates eye and brain vessels [45] and is therefore also used to study the cerebral perfusion reserve. Many decades ago, we and others found that acetazolamide can improve the visual fields in certain glaucoma patients [46]. Later, we realized that these patients had FS. With acetazolamide, we can determine whether some of the visual field defects are still reversible. Acetazolamide is rarely used as a long-term therapy because of its side effects.

CAIs used locally, such as dorzolamides, have fewer systematic side effects and also improve blood flow, albeit to a lesser extent than acetazolamides [47]. Therefore, they are ideal for glaucoma patients with FS despite their limited ability to lower IOP.

4.2.8. NO Donators

NO donators are theoretically interesting for treatment of FS. Unfortunately, very little research has been done on the use of such drugs in FS patients. Nevertheless, it has already been shown that nitrates can lower RVP (ARVO Annual Meeting Abstract, 2017).

Calcium-L-methylfolate (the biologically active form of folic acid) not only reduces homocysteine but also increases NO production via activation of the NO synthetase, thereby improving vasodilatation. Vitamin supplementation containing L-methylfolate (Ocufolin® forte) has shown promise. It improves diabetic and hypertensive retinopathy [48], conjunctival microcirculation [49], and retinal blood flow in diabetes patients [50]. Ocufolin® forte has been studied little in glaucoma so far. However, we already know that it reduces elevated retinal venous pressure (in preparation).

4.2.9. Antioxidants

We have already emphasized the importance of oxidative stress and antioxidant nutrition in the nutritional recommendations section. Although oxidative stress can occur systemically, local stress in certain organs and cells is even more important. Even within a cell, oxidative stress is often very localized (e.g., in mitochondria). Therefore, we cannot simply reduce all oxidative stress with any antioxidant. For example, in patients with glaucoma, stress occurs mainly (but not only) in the mitochondria of the axons in the optic nerve head. A balanced varied antioxidative diet contains molecules that reach these sites. The situation is different with antioxidative supplementation or therapy. Here, one must be purposefully selective. Ginkgo biloba, for example, has proven to reach the mitochondria of axons and exert their effect there. Other molecules are also promising and are currently being investigated (e.g., vitamin supplementation containing calcium-L-methylfolate). Doses of any antioxidants that are too high should imperatively be avoided because all antioxidants become prooxidants if the concentration in the body is too high.

4.3. Pharmaceutical Treatment of Systemic Hypotension

Arterial hypertension (high BP) is a frequent and well-known risk factor for many diseases. Correspondingly, there are also many treatment options. Less well known, however, is the fact that arterial hypotension (low BP), one of the leading FS symptoms [51,52], can also be a risk factor. Many studies have shown that low BP, increased BP fluctuations, nocturnal dips of BP, and orthostatic hypotension increase the risk of occurrence and progression of glaucomatous damage [53]. We are therefore often asked by patients what they can do to increase BP.

We always start with simple interventions, such as increasing salt (sodium chloride) intake mostly in the evening and physical activity. To better control the intake of additional salt, the pharmacist can prepare salt tablets. If the salt is poorly tolerated, it can be taken together with tomato juice.

FS patients should avoid certain drugs as much as possible. Many medications, especially sleeping pills and sedatives, have a side effect of lowering BP. The advantages and disadvantages of such treatments must therefore be weighed against each other.

In the case of orthostatic hypotension, we recommend that patients get up slowly in the morning. We recommend support stockings for people who are in a profession that requires them to stand (or sit) for a long time.

If all this is not sufficient, pharmacological therapy may be considered in rare cases. Although vasoconstrictive drugs are relatively often prescribed for this purpose, they reduce blood flow to the eyes despite an increase in BP and are therefore counterproductive in such cases.

We have had good experiences with a very low dose of fludrocortisone (2×0.1 mg per week) [54]. Fludrocortisone is a mineralocorticoid and not a glucocorticoid and therefore has fewer side effects than glucocorticoids.

The good news is that BP does not necessarily need to be totally normalized. In patients with severe hypotension, even a slight increase in BP leads to significantly better vascular regulation.

5. What Does This All Mean in Practice?

We already mentioned that not all people with FS need treatment. The good news is that very different FS-related phenomena usually respond to treatment in parallel. We found that FS patients often display the following disease signs at the same time: NTG [7], disturbed autoregulation of ocular blood flow [55], increased retinal venous pressure [14], and optic nerve compartment syndrome [3,56]. In most cases, treatment with a low dose of nifedipine (mostly combined with magnesium) simultaneously improved the regulation of retinal vessels, reduced RVP [57], and reduced optic nerve compartment syndrome [56].

How do we ensure that a chosen therapy works? In the end, the main criterion is organ and system function (e.g., the visual field in glaucoma). However, in most cases, we would like to see the effect more quickly. There are subjective criteria. If, for example, a patient notices that his hands have become warmer, then we are very likely on the right track.

However, there are also helpful objective parameters. A reduction of the RVP or an improved reaction of the retinal vessels to flickering light or a shortening of the flow standstill after cold provocation in nailfold capillary microscopy shows us that the treatment has a positive effect.

6. Conclusions

If glaucoma damage progresses despite normal or normalized IOP, then vascular factors are usually involved [6]. One of the vascular factors is primary vascular dysregulation [3], the main component of FS. There are several reasons why FS may be a risk factor for glaucoma damage. Patients with FS are more likely to have (a) impaired autoregulation [55], (b) low blood pressure [4,51], (c) high retinal venous pressure [14], and (d) activated astrocytes [58].

Therefore, we can expect that treatment of FS will improve the prognosis of glaucoma. However, this is yet to be proven in controlled long-term studies.

Author Contributions: K.K. and J.F. wrote, read, and approved the submitted version of the manuscript. All authors have read and agreed to the published version of the manuscript.

Funding: External funding did not support the writing of this publication.

Institutional Review Board Statement: Not applicable.

Informed Consent Statement: Not applicable.

Data Availability Statement: Not applicable.

Conflicts of Interest: The authors declare no conflict of interest.

References

1. Konieczka, K.; Ritch, R.; Traverso, C.E.; Kim, D.M.; Kook, M.S.; Gallino, A.; Golubnitschaja, O.; Erb, C.; Reitsamer, H.A.; Kida, T.; et al. Flammer syndrome. *EPMA J.* **2014**, *5*, 1–7. [CrossRef]
2. Flammer, J.; Konieczka, K.; Bruno, R.M.; Virdis, A.; Flammer, A.J.; Taddei, S. The eye and the heart. *Eur. Heart J.* **2013**, *34*, 1270–1278. [CrossRef]
3. Flammer, J.; Konieczka, K.; Flammer, A.J. The primary vascular dysregulation syndrome: Implications for eye diseases. *EPMA J.* **2013**, *4*, 1–33. [CrossRef]
4. Konieczka, K.; Flammer, J. Phenomenology and Clinical Relevance of the Flammer Syndrome. *Klin. Mon. Fur Augenheilkd.* **2016**, *233*, 1331–1336. [CrossRef]
5. Flammer, J.; Konieczka, K. The discovery of the Flammer syndrome: A historical and personal perspective. *EPMA J.* **2017**, *8*, 75–97. [CrossRef] [PubMed]
6. Flammer, J.; Orgul, S.; Costa, V.P.; Orzalesi, N.; Krieglstein, G.K.; Serra, L.M.; Renard, J.P.; Stefansson, E. The impact of ocular blood flow in glaucoma. *Prog. Retin. Eye Res.* **2002**, *21*, 359–393. [CrossRef]
7. Konieczka, K.; Choi, H.J.; Koch, S.; Fankhauser, F.; Schoetzau, A.; Kim, D.M. Relationship between normal tension glaucoma and Flammer syndrome. *EPMA J.* **2017**, *8*, 111–117. [CrossRef] [PubMed]

8. Konieczka, K.; Erb, C. Diseases potentially related to Flammer syndrome. *EPMA J.* **2017**, *8*, 327–332. [CrossRef] [PubMed]
9. Konieczka, K.; Frankl, S.; Todorova, M.G.; Henrich, P.B. Unstable oxygen supply and glaucoma. *Klin. Mon. Fur Augenheilkd.* **2014**, *231*, 121–126. [CrossRef] [PubMed]
10. Saner, H.; Wurbel, H.; Mahler, F.; Flammer, J.; Gasser, P. Microvasculatory evaluation of vasospastic syndromes. *Adv. Exp. Med. Biol.* **1987**, *220*, 215–218.
11. Nicolela, M.T.; Ferrier, S.N.; Morrison, C.A.; Archibald, M.L.; LeVatte, T.L.; Wallace, K.; Chauhan, B.C.; LeBlanc, R.P. Effects of cold-induced vasospasm in glaucoma: The role of endothelin-1. *Investig. Ophthalmol. Vis. Sci.* **2003**, *44*, 2565–2572. [CrossRef] [PubMed]
12. Terelak-Borys, B.; Grabska-Liberek, I.; Schoetzau, A.; Konieczka, K. Transient visual field impairment after cold provocation in glaucoma patients with Flammer syndrome. *Restor. Neurol. Neurosci.* **2019**, *37*, 31–39. [CrossRef]
13. Sabel, B.A.; Lehnigk, L. Is Mental Stress the Primary Cause of Glaucoma? *Klin. Monbl. Augenheilkd.* **2021**, *238*, 132–145.
14. Fang, L.; Baertschi, M.; Mozaffarieh, M. The effect of flammer-syndrome on retinal venous pressure. *BMC Ophthalmol.* **2014**, *14*, 1–5. [CrossRef] [PubMed]
15. Mustur, D.; Vahedian, Z.; Bovet, J.; Mozaffarieh, M. Retinal venous pressure measurements in patients with Flammer syndrome and metabolic syndrome. *EPMA J.* **2017**, *8*, 339–344. [CrossRef] [PubMed]
16. Josifova, T.; Fankhauser, F.; Konieczka, K. Flammer Syndrome, A Potential Risk Factor for Central Serous Chorioretinopathy? *Biomed. J. Sci. Tech. Res.* **2020**, *24*, 18115–18119. [CrossRef]
17. Prunte, C.; Flammer, J. Choroidal capillary and venous congestion in central serous chorioretinopathy. *Am. J. Ophthalmol.* **1996**, *121*, 26–34. [CrossRef]
18. Konieczka, K.; Gugleta, K. *Glaukom*; Hans Huber: Berlin, Germany, 2015.
19. Heitmar, R.; Gherghel, D.; Armstrong, R.; Cubbidge, R.; Hosking, S. The effect of voluntary fasting and dehydration on flicker-induced retinal vascular dilation in a healthy individual: A case report. *J. Med. Case Rep.* **2008**, *2*, 1–7. [CrossRef]
20. Mozaffarieh, M.; Schoetzau, A.; Sauter, M.; Grieshaber, M.; Orgul, S.; Golubnitschaja, O.; Flammer, J. Comet assay analysis of single-stranded DNA breaks in circulating leukocytes of glaucoma patients. *Mol. Vis.* **2008**, *14*, 1584–1588.
21. Erb, C.; Heinke, M. Oxidative stress in primary open-angle glaucoma. *Front. Biosci.* **2011**, *3*, 1524–1533. [CrossRef]
22. Mozaffarieh, M.; Grieshaber, M.C.; Orgul, S.; Flammer, J. The potential value of natural antioxidative treatment in glaucoma. *Surv. Ophthalmol.* **2008**, *53*, 479–505. [CrossRef]
23. Flammer, J.; Mozaffarieh, M.; Bebie, H. *Basic Sciences in Ophthalmology*; Springer: Berlin/Heidelberg, Germany, 2013.
24. Konieczka, K.; Flammer, J.; Erb, C. Diseases associated with Flammer Syndrome: An Update. *Biomed. J. Sci. Tech. Res.* **2020**, *25*, 19098–19103. [CrossRef]
25. Bojinova, R.I.; Konieczka, K.; Meyer, P.; Todorova, M.G. The trilateral link between anaesthesia, perioperative visual loss and Flammer syndrome. *BMC Anesthesiol.* **2016**, *16*, 1–10. [CrossRef]
26. Bojinova, R.I.; Konieczka, K.; Todorova, M.G. Unilateral Loss of Vision after Spinal Surgery in a Patient with Flammer Syndrome. *Klin. Mon. Fur Augenheilkd.* **2016**, *233*, 429–431. [CrossRef] [PubMed]
27. Konieczka, K.; Koch, S.; Hauenstein, D.; Chackathayil, T.N.; Binggeli, T.; Schoetzau, A.; Flammer, J. Effects of the Glaucoma Drugs Latanoprost and Brimonidine on Corneal Temperature. *Transl. Vis. Sci. Technol.* **2019**, *8*, 47. [CrossRef]
28. Meyer, P.; Lang, M.G.; Flammer, J.; Luscher, T.F. Effects of calcium channel blockers on the response to endothelin-1, bradykinin and sodium nitroprusside in porcine ciliary arteries. *Exp. Eye Res.* **1995**, *60*, 505–510. [CrossRef]
29. Lang, M.G.; Zhu, P.; Meyer, P.; Noll, G.; Haefliger, I.O.; Flammer, J.; Luscher, T.F. Amlodipine and benazeprilat differently affect the responses to endothelin-1 and bradykinin in porcine ciliary arteries: Effects of a low and high dose combination. *Curr. Eye Res.* **1997**, *16*, 208–213. [CrossRef]
30. Teuchner, B.; Orgul, S.; Ulmer, H.; Haufschild, T.; Flammer, J. Reduced thirst in patients with a vasospastic syndrome. *Acta Ophthalmol. Scand.* **2004**, *82*, 738–740. [CrossRef]
31. Gass, A.; Flammer, J.; Linder, L.; Romerio, S.C.; Gasser, P.; Haefeli, W.E. Inverse correlation between endothelin-1-induced peripheral microvascular vasoconstriction and blood pressure in glaucoma patients. *Graefe's Arch. Clin. Exp. Ophthalmol. Albrecht Graefes Arch. Klin. Exp. Ophthalmol.* **1997**, *235*, 634–638. [CrossRef] [PubMed]
32. Flammer, J.; Drance, S.M. Effect of acetazolamide on the differential threshold. *Arch. Ophthalmol.* **1983**, *101*, 1378–1380. [CrossRef]
33. Guthauser, U.; Flammer, J.; Mahler, F. The relationship between digital and ocular vasospasm. *Graefe's Arch. Clin. Exp. Ophthalmol. Albrecht Graefes Arch. Klin. Exp. Ophthalmol.* **1988**, *226*, 224–226. [CrossRef] [PubMed]
34. Gugleta, K.; Orgul, S.; Hasler, P.; Flammer, J. Circulatory response to blood gas perturbations in vasospasm. *Investig. Ophthalmol. Vis. Sci.* **2005**, *46*, 3288–3294. [CrossRef] [PubMed]
35. Liu, S.; Araujo, S.V.; Spaeth, G.L.; Katz, L.J.; Smith, M. Lack of effect of calcium channel blockers on open-angle glaucoma. *J. Glaucoma* **1996**, *5*, 187–190. [CrossRef] [PubMed]
36. Riva, C.E.; Cranstoun, S.D.; Petrig, B.L. Effect of decreased ocular perfusion pressure on blood flow and the flicker-induced flow response in the cat optic nerve head. *Microvasc. Res.* **1996**, *52*, 258–269. [CrossRef]
37. Flammer, J.; Konieczka, K. Retinal venous pressure: The role of endothelin. *EPMA J.* **2015**, *6*, 1–12. [CrossRef]
38. Konieczka, K.; Meyer, P.; Schoetzau, A.; Neutzner, A.; Mozaffarieh, M.; Flammer, J. Effect of avosentan (SPP-301) in porcine ciliary arteries. *Curr. Eye Res.* **2011**, *36*, 118–124. [CrossRef]

39. Neumann, T.; Baertschi, M.; Vilser, W.; Drinda, S.; Franz, M.; Bruckmann, A.; Wolf, G.; Jung, C. Retinal vessel regulation at high altitudes1. *Clin. Hemorheol. Microcirc.* **2016**, *63*, 281–292. [CrossRef]
40. Jain, A.; Coffey, C.; Mehrotra, V.; Flammer, J. Endothelin-1 traps as a potential therapeutic tool: From diabetes to beyond? *Drug Discov. Today* **2019**, *24*, 1937–1942. [CrossRef]
41. Dettmann, E.S.; Luscher T.F.; Flammer, J.; Haefliger, I.O. Modulation of endothelin-1-induced contractions by magnesium/calcium in porcine ciliary arteries. *Graefe's Arch. Clin. Exp. Ophthalmol. Albrecht Graefes Arch. Klin. Exp. Ophthalmol.* **1998**, *236*, 47–51. [CrossRef]
42. Gaspar, A.Z.; Gasser, P.; Flammer, J. The influence of magnesium on visual field and peripheral vasospasm in glaucoma. *Ophthalmologica* **1995**, *209*, 11–13. [CrossRef]
43. Grieshaber, M.C.; Flammer, J. Is the medication used to achieve the target intraocular pressure in glaucoma therapy of relevance?—An exemplary analysis on the basis of two beta-blockers. *Prog. Retin. Eye Res.* **2010**, *29*, 79–93. [CrossRef]
44. Shin, S.; Kim, K.J.; Cho, I.J.; Hong, G.R.; Jang, Y.; Chung, N.; Rah, Y.M.; Chang, H.J. Effect of Triflusal on Primary Vascular Dysregulation Compared with Aspirin: A Double-Blind, Randomized, Crossover Trial. *Yonsei Med. J.* **2015**, *56*, 1227–1234. [CrossRef]
45. Petropoulos, I.K.; Pournaras, J.A.; Munoz, J.L.; Pournaras, C.J. Effect of acetazolamide on the optic disc oxygenation in miniature pigs. *Klin. Monbl. Augenheilkd.* **2004**, *221*, 367–370.
46. Flammer, J.; Drance, S.M. Reversibility of a glaucomatous visual field defect after acetazolamide therapy. *Can. J. Ophthalmol.* **1983**, *18*, 139–141.
47. Nagel, E.; Vilser, W.; Lanzl, I. Dorzolamide influences the autoregulation of major retinal vessels caused by artificial intraocular pressure elevation in patients with POAG: A clinical study. *Curr. Eye Res.* **2005**, *30*, 129–137. [CrossRef]
48. Wang, J.; Brown, C.; Shi, C.; Townsend, J.; Gameiro, G.R.; Wang, P.; Jiang, H. Improving diabetic and hypertensive retinopathy with a medical food containing L-methylfolate: A preliminary report. *Eye Vis.* **2019**, *6*, 1–11. [CrossRef]
49. Liu, Z.; Jiang, H.; Townsend, J.H.; Wang, J. Improved conjunctival microcirculation in diabetic retinopathy patients with MTHFR polymorphisms after Ocufolin Administration. *Microvasc. Res.* **2020**, *132*, 104066. [CrossRef] [PubMed]
50. Schmidl, D.; Howorka, K.; Szegedi, S.; Stjepanek, K.; Puchner, S.; Bata, A.; Scheschy, U.; Aschinger, G.; Werkmeister, R.M.; Schmetterer, L.; et al. A pilot study to assess the effect of a three-month vitamin supplementation containing L-methylfolate on systemic homocysteine plasma concentrations and retinal blood flow in patients with diabetes. *Mol. Vis.* **2020**, *26*, 326–333.
51. Gherghel, D.; Orgul, S.; Gugleta, K.; Flammer, J. Retrobulbar blood flow in glaucoma patients with nocturnal over-dipping in systemic blood pressure. *Am. J. Ophthalmol.* **2001**, *132*, 641–647. [CrossRef]
52. Binggeli, T.; Schoetzau, A.; Konieczka, K. In glaucoma patients, low blood pressure is accompanied by vascular dysregulation. *EPMA J.* **2018**, *9*, 387–391. [CrossRef] [PubMed]
53. Kaiser, H.J.; Flammer, J.; Graf, T.; Stumpfig, D. Systemic blood pressure in glaucoma patients. *Graefe's Arch. Clin. Exp. Ophthalmol. Albrecht Graefes Arch. Klin. Exp. Ophthalmol.* **1993**, *231*, 677–680. [CrossRef] [PubMed]
54. Gugleta, K.; Orgul, S.; Stumpfig, D.; Dubler, B.; Flammer, J. Fludrocortisone in the treatment of systemic hypotension in primary open-angle glaucoma patients. *Int. Ophthalmol.* **1999**, *23*, 25–30. [CrossRef] [PubMed]
55. Gherghel, D.; Orgul, S.; Dubler, B.; Lubeck, P.; Gugleta, K.; Flammer, J. Is vascular regulation in the central retinal artery altered in persons with vasospasm? *Arch. Ophthalmol.* **1999**, *117*, 1359–1362. [CrossRef]
56. Konieczka, K.; Todorova, M.G.; Bojinova, R.I.; Binggeli, T.; Chackathayil, T.N.; Flammer, J. Unexpected Effect of Calcium Channel Blockers on the Optic Nerve Compartment Syndrome. *Klin. Mon. Augenheilkd.* **2016**, *233*, 387–390. [CrossRef] [PubMed]
57. Fang, L.; Turtschi, S.; Mozaffarieh, M. The effect of nifedipine on retinal venous pressure of glaucoma patients with the Flammer-Syndrome. *Graefe's Arch. Clin. Exp. Ophthalmol. Albrecht Graefes Arch. Klin. Exp. Ophthalmol.* **2015**, *253*, 935–939. [CrossRef]
58. Grieshaber, M.C.; Orgul, S.; Schoetzau, A.; Flammer, J. Relationship between retinal glial cell activation in glaucoma and vascular dysregulation. *J. Glaucoma* **2007**, *16*, 215–219. [CrossRef] [PubMed]

MDPI
St. Alban-Anlage 66
4052 Basel
Switzerland
www.mdpi.com

Journal of Clinical Medicine Editorial Office
E-mail: jcm@mdpi.com
www.mdpi.com/journal/jcm

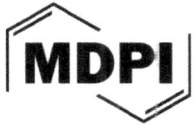

Disclaimer/Publisher's Note: The statements, opinions and data contained in all publications are solely those of the individual author(s) and contributor(s) and not of MDPI and/or the editor(s). MDPI and/or the editor(s) disclaim responsibility for any injury to people or property resulting from any ideas, methods, instructions or products referred to in the content.

www.ingramcontent.com/pod-product-compliance
Lightning Source LLC
LaVergne TN
LVHW070044120526
838202LV00101B/425